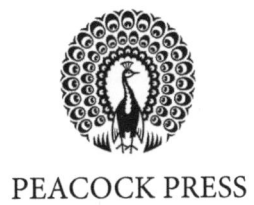

PEACOCK PRESS

Isaac Milburn the Northumbrian Bonesetter 1794–1886
by Bruce Burns

ISBN: 978-1-914934-34-6

Published 2022 by: Peacock Press, Scout Bottom Farm, Mytholmroyd, Hebden Bridge HX7 5JS (UK). 01422 882751.

Book design by www.SiPat.co.uk

All rights reserved. No part of this publication may be reproduced, stored or transmitted in any form or by any means electronically or mechanically, by photocopying, recording, scanning or otherwise, without the permission of the copyright owners. © Peacock Press

ISAAC MILBURN

The Northumbrian Bonesetter
1794–1886

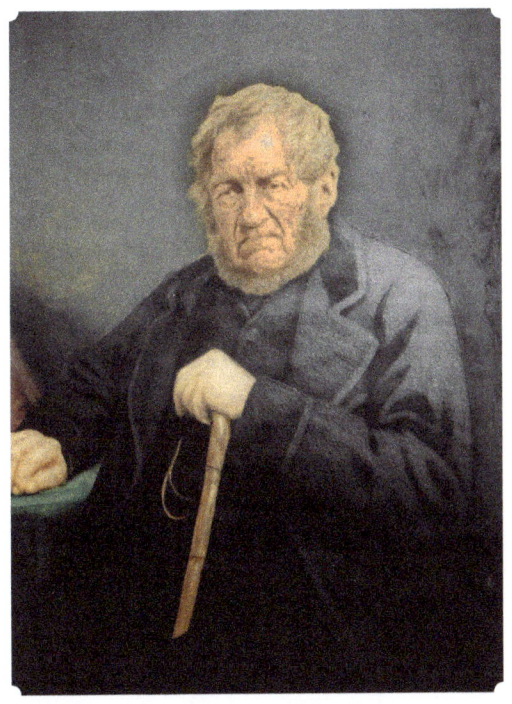

ONE MAN'S INCREDIBLE STORY

From gamekeeper at Wallington
Hall to Royal bonesetter.

His amazing life story. Whisky smuggling,
poaching and a gunpowder plot. A controversial
figure in the world of medicine.

BY BRUCE BURNS

ISAAC MILBURN: THE NORTHUMBRIAN BONESETTER [1794 - 1886]

CONTENTS

	Introduction	7
1.	The Early Years	11
2.	Smugglers and Poachers	17
3.	Leaving Wallington Hall	29
4.	Isaac's Casebook	41
5.	A Royal Appointment, Gunpowder, Treason and Plot	47
6.	Testimonial	55
7.	Death of Isaac Milburn	61
8.	Controversy	67
9.	Isaac's Legacy	79
10.	Milburn Family Tree	85
11.	Key Dates	89
12.	Surname Cast List	91
	Print References	97
	Photograph Acknowledgements	99
	Glossary	103
	The Author	107

INTRODUCTION

It has been an honour and privilege to be able to research the life of my four times Great Grandfather Isaac Milburn.

The more I have looked into his incredible journey from gamekeeper to treating members of the Royal family the more I have been convinced that this is a story that needs to be told. I have found interesting facts at almost every corner and I am sure there is even more to find. This may only be the start but it is a fascinating glimpse into the life of a bonesetter, a profession that has been rarely recognised and to this day still generates divided opinion upon medical experts.

Newspaper cuttings during his lifetime graphically illustrate his skills. He "would pull into position limbs that had been fractured". This resetting of dislocated and broken limbs and bones would have been a considerably difficult task without the modern-day anaesthetics we now take for granted and where pain is almost eliminated.

A bonesetter in the 19th century may have required the help and strength of others under expert guidance, to manipulate the broken bones back into position. Any errors in procedure could conclude in continuous agony for the patient, misaligned joints, swelling and a whole host of other associated problems. This could ruin the reputation of an unskilled or back street bonesetter.

Testament to the undoubted professional expertise of Isaac Milburn is the fact he was able to be a renowned bonesetter for more than 60 years, lasting until well into his 90s. An incredible rubber stamping of his valued reputation. From humble beginnings in the late 18th century his standing as a bonesetter knew no bounds. From treating the injured throughout Northumberland to what is widely believed to be those of Royal associations.

His work has been recorded in various newspaper articles, letters, books and general hearsay over the centuries. This is an attempt to collate, preserve and enlighten the memory of a man, part of my family, who undoubtedly had immense skill and great character. It has been possible to pull together a rich vein of material to cast a light on Isaac Milburn's renowned resourcefulness.

The portrait on the cover of this book is my earliest encounter with my Great Great Great Great Grandfather. My grandparents, Isaac and Mary Milburn, had it hung on the wall of the spare bedroom of Milburn House, Etal Road, Tweedmouth, where they lived and where I occasionally had sleepovers in my boyhood. It was painted in the late 1800s and it has survived intact over the years.

Despite woodworm and the discarded ornate picture frame, it was handed down by my grandfather to his son Isaac and is now in the possession of his grandson - also called Isaac Milburn to add to the confusion.

I think it was painted when Isaac was aged about 85 and although it used to scare me, just me and him alone in the room, I now believe it captures the character of a gruff looking, tough old man, deep in his thought in his twilight years.

Note the gold chain of his pocket watch which has a Royal connection that you can read about in due course.

I hope my efforts to tell his story are not in vain. I would like to think they help to stimulate further research and possibly be a catalyst for more descendants to step forward and help make the story even richer.

Any proceeds from this publication will be used to ensure his grave and headstone are well maintained in future years.

As always I am indebted to others for their help with his treasure trove of memories. Mary Kipling (PR1) who self-published a short account of a bonesetter's life in the 1960s and was able to speak to some surviving family members and pass on invaluable information that would otherwise have been lost.

Wendy Maltby very kindly gave me permission to reproduce any information published by Mary and her oil painting you see on the back cover. Other contributions have been eagerly retrieved from newspaper articles, books and letters. All of these have been detailed in the reference section.

Many thanks also to my lifelong friends Ron Clarke, Dr Aniela Morawiecki, Keith Ryan and Peter Vousden for their proof reading skills and most helpful suggestions.

His original mode of speech has been retained where possible and definitions of certain words can be found in the glossary.

Chapter 12 includes an A-Z list of people's names and places appearing in this book which may help others researching family history in the Northumberland area.

Place names mentioned in the book are shown on the inside front cover map of Northumberland and a few local maps on other pages which have initially been typed in bold text as an easy reference guide for those readers unfamiliar with the area.

I would dearly like to hear from anyone who may have even more information about Isaac Milburn. Please contact me by email *bburns.ecosse@virgin.net*.

ISAAC MILBURN: THE NORTHUMBRIAN BONESETTER 1794 - 1886

CHAPTER 1
THE EARLY YEARS

Isaac was born 6th April 1794 at the little group of buildings at Throphill in the parish of Mitford some five miles west of Morpeth. His mother was Elizabeth and his father William was a country joiner, a cartwright who would appear to have had the ability to work on any little mechanical job required by the agricultural and rural population among whom they lived. Isaac had a brother Christopher and two sisters Mary and Jane. It is said William had the skill and nerve to set a broken limb and replace an erring joint when extremity was required and Isaac got his first taste for what became his business. As a young lad Isaac followed his father's trade in the little workshop adjoining a byre in Throphill but his interests lay in another direction.

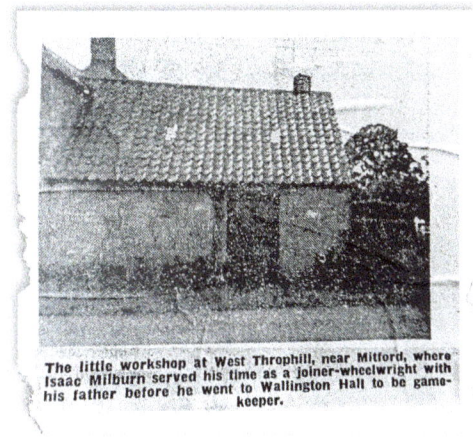
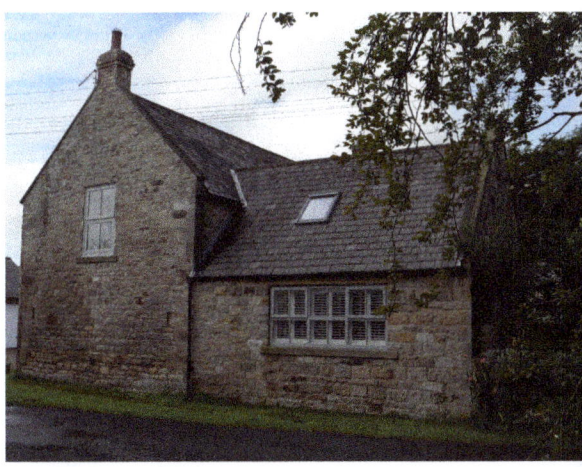

The little workshop at West Throphill, near Mitford, where Isaac Milburn served his time as a joiner-wheelwright with his father before he went to Wallington Hall to be gamekeeper.

1, left. Workshop. 2, right. The restored property in 2021.

Quitting the work-bench he entered a "gentleman's service" as a valet, at Wallington Hall and for some years was employed in that capacity before becoming gamekeeper for the estate. Wallington Hall owned by the Trevelyan family is an impressive country house estate with over 100 acres of farmland, woodland, ornamental lakes, lawns and a walled garden. Isaac's first boss was Sir John Trevelyan the 4th Baronet 1734 – 1828. Sir John was a member of an ancient Cornish family and a British conservative politician from 1777 to 1796. He inherited Wallington Hall with other Northumbrian estates from his wife's uncle in 1777 and it was said that Sir John was one of Isaac's early patients. The property and estate have been managed by the National Trust since 1942, and are open to the public.

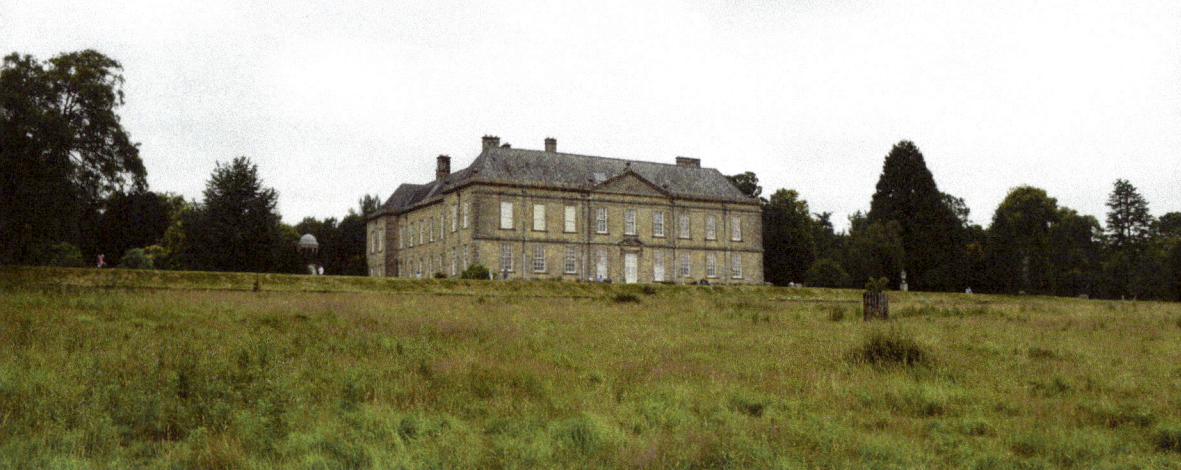

3. Wallington Hall.

Isaac married on the 12th April 1823 at the age of 29 Elizabeth Thornton who was five years younger and originally from Battle Bridge some 5 miles west of Alnwick. The couple lived in one of the estate properties called Bolt Cottage, a short distance north of the main house. They had three children, Jane born 1824, William in 1827 and Robert 1836, all born at Wallington according to the census records. Bolt Cottage is now available as a beautiful refurbished holiday let from the National Trust with some of the original features such as the stone fireplace and ceiling beams being retained. Interestingly the internal staircase has a wooden balustrade which was removed from Wallington Hall in 1740 when the hall was being refurbished.

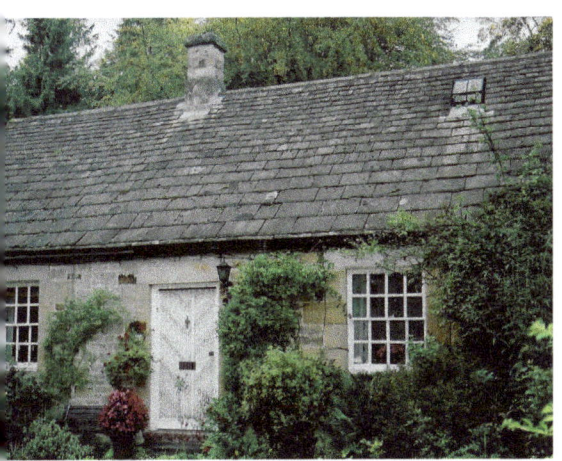 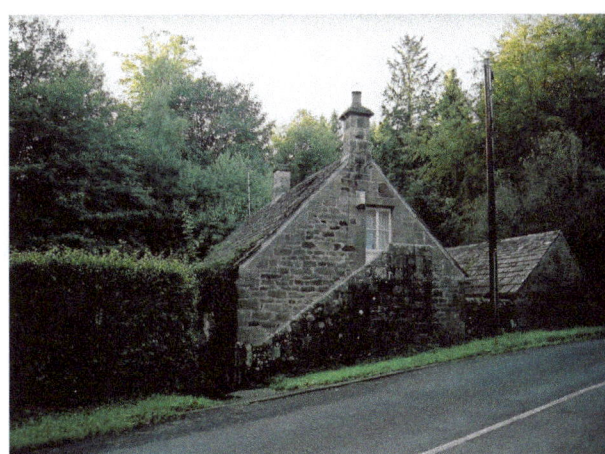

4a / 4b. Bolt Cottage.

This now all looks very idyllic and welcoming but life as a gamekeeper would have been less sumptuous in an environment we would now find a bit shocking and cruel. One of the gamekeeper's duties would be to catch rabbits by means of ferrets and nets in order to minimise crop damage and provide a source of meat. Isaac would pick up a live rabbit and methodically put out first one joint then another. This would be repeated until he had a number of the powerless animals lying inactive, temporarily deprived of their ability to move, only to have the satisfaction of subsequently replacing the dislocated joints and watch the timid creatures scamper off when returned from their helpless condition. Such tales as these have been told of many rural bonesetters. Another bonesetter from the south west of Scotland had an extensive reputation as a boy for manipulations on the poultry and smaller four-footed animals of every farm where his father was employed as a ploughman with a daring freedom.

Mary Kipling says as part of Isaac's education "dead rabbits were hung up until the maggots dropped from them in order to feed the pheasants, he took the bones, cleaned them and practised his bone setting". Breaking bones and understanding the joints of dead animals would therefore have been a way in which Isaac developed an early basic knowledge of anatomy and learned an important aspect of the bonesetter's trade.

The earliest documented mention of Isaac is in "The local historians tablebook of remarkable occurrences Vol 4 by Moses Aaron Richardson" (PR2) who wrote "Isaac Milburn gamekeeper to Sir John Trevelyan of Wallington, fell in with a flight of 23 swans of which by discharge of his double-barrelled shotgun he killed six. Two others fell but escaped under favour of darkness the largest weighed 17 pounds". This tale sets the date as pre 1828, in Sir John's lifetime.

A warning that most, particularly pet owners, will find this next tale from the 1830s even more uncomfortable reading!

Wallington Hall's next owner was Sir John Trevelyan the 5th Baronet. His son was Edward Spencer Trevelyan, and Isaac was his right-hand man on the shooting moor. A book entitled "Memories of Wallington Hall" written by Edward Keith in 1937 (PR3) mentions a fellow estate worker of the time called Codling whose surname appears in a number of early census records, one of which is a coachman living in Wallington Hall cottage. He recounts that Isaac would "pick up a dog pretending to fondle it on his knee and when put down it would lie howling on the ground. Powerless, it's shoulders had been slipped off or its thighs put out of joint, only to be seized again and the damage quickly remedied, so expert became his fingers in manipulating man and beast to dislocate the leg of a gundog and all around would watch it lie motionless whimpering until Isaac put it back into place and off it would run." Codling talked about him "with great admiration as a man though he lamented his cruelty".

Edward Keith was a gardener at Wallington Hall from 1882 – 1933 and his book is about recollections of conversations with Sir George Otto Trevelyan – the Wallington Hall owner 1886 – 1928.

I'm not quite sure how to summarise his actions or even attempt to defend them as they certainly would be condemned by today's standards. Some might say he was a showman in front of an audience and others might claim that these were all part of a crude but necessary self-teaching process before working with humans.

They were certainly different times, some two hundred years ago, when killing animals and living off the land in the countryside was part of rural life, in order to survive. People were much more hardened to such practices. Some fortunate families living on the Wallington Hall estate in Cambo, Close Houses and the Dovecot would each have a piece of land attached to their cottage and they would rely on a cow and a pig as their main source of food. It would have been common for country folk to watch pigs, sheep, hens and cattle being slaughtered in their back yard. This would then be prepared locally, possibly salted and stored in a barrel in order to put food on the table and survive. This practice would eventually die out as estate owners reclaimed the land, and one example of change was that tea eventually replaced cowmilk as the main family beverage, much to the detriment of their children's health. Even my grandparents in the 1930s were keeping a few pigs in a large garden or farm setting and would tell tales of dispatching them with a large hammer and a sharp knife. So practices and attitudes have certainly changed over time and I think we need to bear this in mind when judging how bonesetters living in the countryside learnt their trade.

We first start to get an impression of how Isaac's bone setting skills began to spread around the nearby villages and towns, while he was working at

Wallington Hall from an article in the Newcastle Courant in 1879 (PR4). The unknown writer states "at first his practice of the bone setting art was undertaken solely from benevolent and neighbourly motives and his patients were the unfortunates who lived within a few miles of his cottage, his services being rendered without fee or reward beyond the satisfaction of having benefited a suffering acquaintance, and that peculiar gratification afforded by the consciousness of having performed an act that no known equal and few superiors could have done."

A neighbour of Isaac's recalled vividly two of his earliest cases. A young lad who lived with his father, had the misfortune while playing to put his wrist out. His father took him to see Isaac at the Dovecot and almost simultaneously arrived a man with a dislocated knee – helpless and suffering acute agony. The older sufferer was taken in hand first, and the boy with dread and fear watched the process, whereby the confident and powerful gamekeeper replaced the joint in its socket. At the end of a short operation, the crippled man stood up and used the limb. The boys turn then came, and with a dexterity that surprised him his wrist was put in, and in his own words "in an instant I was translated from purgatory to paradise"

By such cases as these Isaac gradually acquired experience and confidence, and each new incidence of success carried his reputation for skill and cleverness over an ever widening area.

Here follows a few more cases:

The Strong man

There is a story of a very strong man who went to Isaac to be treated for a hip joint injury.

It seems the patient was enduring great pain, and the prospect of greater – which might be many degrees more intense though of brief duration – made him fidgety, ill to manage and difficult to get him into the correct position. Isaac worked on him for an unusually long period of time and eventually with somewhat expressive language to assert his authority and compel him to get ready. In almost a twinkling of an eye the injury was repaired. Recovering from his amazement the man looked up and said:

> "its *dyeun noo*, Isaac"

> "*aye*" said Milburn with one of his special though somewhat inelegant expletives

> "its dyeun but you're a great *luggish*"

I'm not absolutely certain what luggish means but probably you are a bit of whimp considering your strength and stature.

South Northumberland Girl

By way of contrast with the above example the next two cases illustrate fairly the gentler side of Isaac's character which could just as easily be judiciously brought into action. A little girl – a mere child - from the far south of Northumberland, who had in a way unknown to her parents received some injury to her arm or shoulder. For a fortnight the family doctor wrought on with it causing the little one no end of pain.

On the advice of a relative she was carried off to Isaac, who by genial tact, diverted her attention away from him and herself, and she was unaware of his doing anything to her. He had with a hand as gentle as that of a woman, found the seat of the injury and by one sharp movement replaced the tender joint, enabling her to once more embrace her overjoyed mother.

J.A.J. Devonshire

The other was a boy with initials J.A.J from Devonshire, who dislocated one of his big toes whilst bathing at Whitley Bay. It was thought that it was a simple sprain and for some time was treated as such at home. After a delay of some weeks he went to Isaac, who as soon as it came the lad's turn, engaged him in conversation about where it happened, where he belonged to, what he was doing, and just as he had him puzzled with what he was going to be, a clear distinct crack and a twitch of sharp pain told him the joint had been returned back to its proper place.

Before he left Wallington Hall his services were sought after by persons far beyond the district in which he lived, and even gentlefolks did not think it beneath their dignity to have their fractures reduced by the gamekeeper at Wallington.

Historically bonesetters would treat fractures and manipulate joints. After the dissolution of the monasteries in the 16th century monks and nuns with knowledge of medicine became healers and bonesetters. Many bonesetters were non-religious, self-taught and their skills passed down from family to family. By the 19th century bone-setting became common practice and was less expensive than the growing number of trained physicians who became a regulated body by the 1858 Medical Act.

CHAPTER 2

SMUGGLERS AND POACHERS

This chapter is a fascinating insight into smuggling at Wallington Hall in Northumberland. Of course Isaac was involved and in a series of letters by Edward Spencer Trevelyan to his mother in 1830 tell us all about it. We later hear about life at Wallington Hall around 1830 and poaching. The letters were reprinted in a booklet published by Frank Graham (PR5).

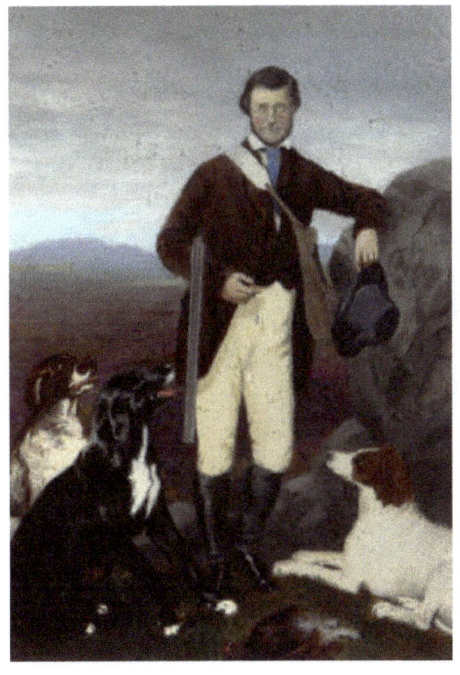

I think it best to reprint the letters in their entirety, with some word explanations in italics, as this gives a greater understanding of the smuggling and also illustrates the courageous and caring side of Isaac's nature as well as his medical skills at the age of 36.

5. Edward Spencer Trevelyan. A small full-length oil portrait of Edward Spencer Trevelyan (1805-1854) with a gun resting over his right arm and surrounded by hunting dogs is displayed at Wallington Hall by the National Trust.

Wallington, June 12th, Sunday 1830 Newcastle-on-Tyne

My dear Mother

I have had a very busy time of it for the last 28 hours. About 1 o clock yesterday a man rode up to the front door and rang the bell. He was covered in blood and mud and could not keep his legs when he dismounted. I got him washed and as soon as he could speak, I learnt that he was one of 3 persons connected with the Excise, who had been engaged with 2 Irish smugglers a short way south of Little Harle Guide Post (somewhere between Old and New Deanham) and that he had left his two companions lying dead or nearly so, on the road. I immediately sent Creighton and his man to assist them and they were brought here in a dreadful state. The heads of all three were almost entire wounds from bludgeons, the skull bared in many places; one of them Mr Griffiths of Alnwick, stabbed in the back and side; his cheek cut with a knife from the eye to the chin; and a stab which had evidently been aimed at the throat, but had taken effect a little higher – 6 of his teeth were knocked out and his upper lip hanging by a skin and his left arm disabled. I got the blood washed partly from their heads and faces and clapped acres of diachylum over their wounds and with assistance of the women got them to bed.

I sent Charles on the Excise Collector's horse in pursuit of the doctor and Isaac Milburn and John Lawes well-armed in immediate pursuit of the Smugglers – directing them to ride straight away and not to poke about the place where the attack was made. I sent Wilkinson and all the footmen about the place to search the immediate neighbourhood in case of their being concealed and dispatched Mr Winshap after Milburn and Lawes, as, in case the smugglers making straight away, foot people would be of little avail. I told Isaac to call at Capheaton on his way and communicate with Sir John Swinburne, the local Magistrate, supposing that, as he has a stable full of horses, he would of course employ them and his men to assist in the pursuit – but he did no such thing and did not offer any assistance.

In the mean-time Mr Winship and Lawes had joined and got a clue which led them to the top of Shaftoe Crags from which place they viewed two Smugglers going over the fields near Harnham, galloped after them, dodged at their heels, till Isaac with his gun

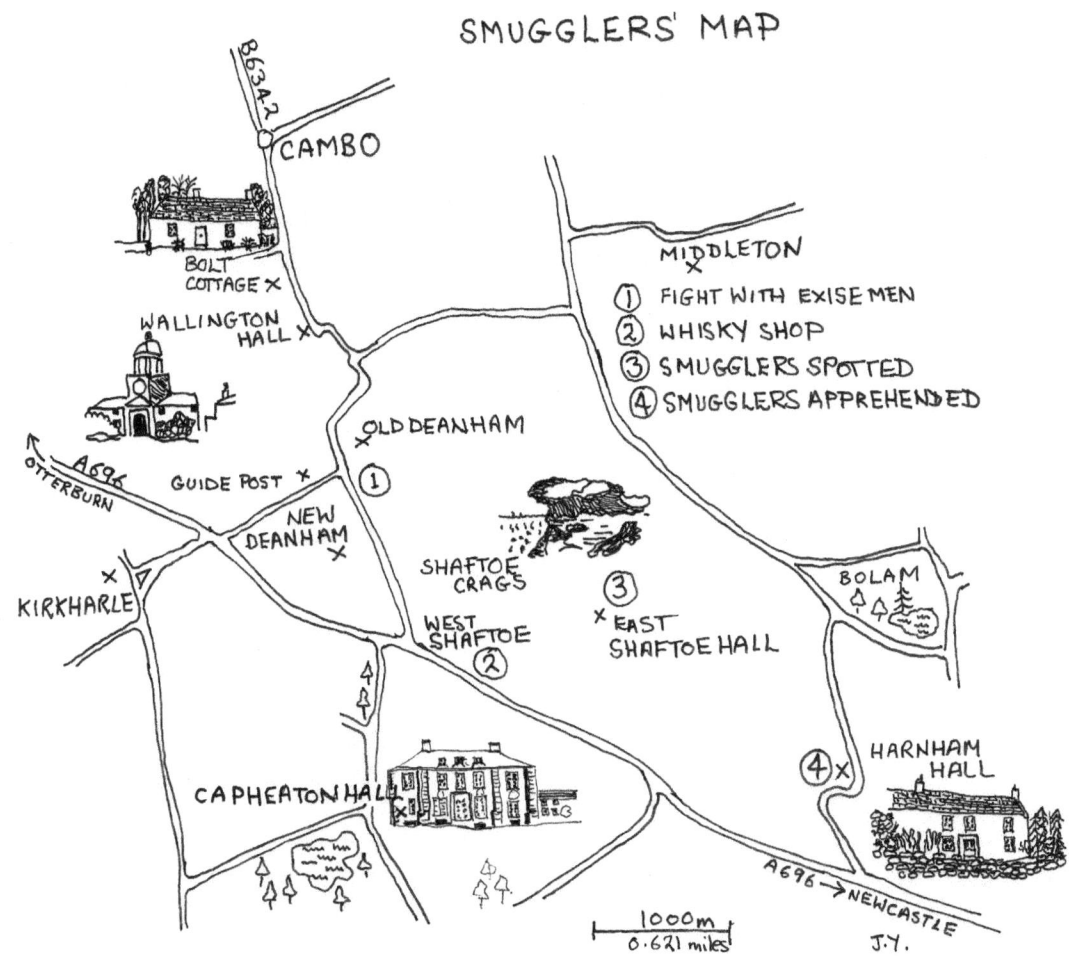

6. Map of the area showing the main roads.

and other assistance came up, when the men surrendered, not without some vaporing. One of them carried an oak stick which was very bloody. Both of them were wounded in the head and had much blood about their clothes. They were taken to Capheaton, but Sir John, with his usual ignorance of Magisterial powers, refused to commit them without examining the Excisemen, though circumstances were far more than sufficiently strong to have warranted their committal, on suspicion. Accordingly the Smugglers were sent here and followed by Sir John in Pott's chaise.

How I laughed when I saw the immense chest of papers, and Burns Justice handed out of the chaise. Sir John after a vast deal of fiddle-faddle and blundering, at last, with Winship's assistance, succeeded in executing the warrant. The Excisemen were not in a fit state to undergo examination, but sufficiently identified the men; and Sir John when they are somewhat recovered, is to come and take their depositions at length. The smugglers were sent to Morpeth Gaol forthwith, guided by the Morpeth Supervisors, for whom an express had been sent, in order that, if we did not catch the Men the Board might take what steps they chose for their apprehension. They had evidently left the men under the idea that they were killed and so unable to give an alarm, so they had not hurried away much and had carried their whisky to within a short distance of the place where they were taken; it was found concealed in a hedge. This, one of the men confessed on his road to Morpeth and said they had no fear of being taken.

They might easily have hid in some of the whin covers about Shaftoe and attempted an escape by night.

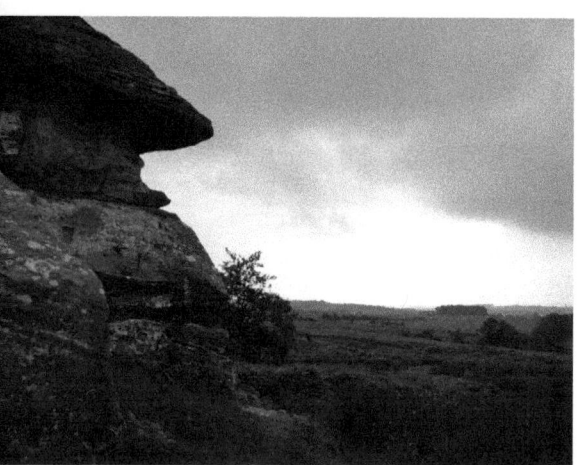
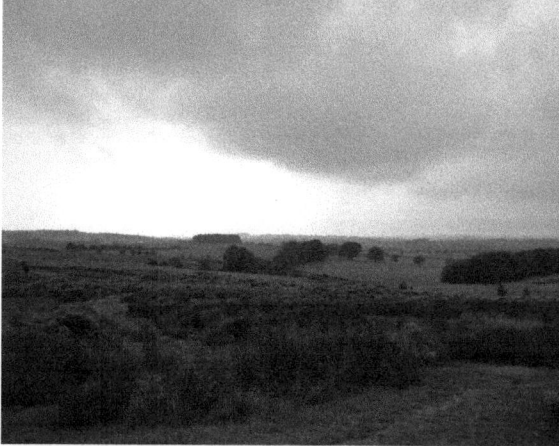

7. Shaftoe Crags.

The Morpeth Supervisor returned this morning, and brought Mr. Hawdon (Surgeon). Griffiths whose wounds I have already described, is in great danger. There is a cudgel wound 4 inches long at the back of his head, which laid the skull bare – and a similar wound of less extent in the forehead – fortunately no fracture of the head. Evans, Collector of Excise for the county, a situation of some importance, had a cudgel wound at the back of the head, and down to the skull, 5 inches long; left eye bunged up, and eyebrow nearly cut off.

He is not out of danger. The third Mr. Cooper, son of an Alderman of York, is least hurt, though he has 6 wounds at the back of the head, two of them to the bone and one bad wound to the forehead. They will not be able to be moved for some days, under the best circumstances. Isaac Milburn's services have proved very valuable. He is a much better operator than Orr, in dressing their wounds, bleeding etc and has had to shave all their heads. Orr, Isaac, myself, John Codling and Richardson, were busy for 3 hours yesterday evening in dressing their wounds. We did not shave them till this morning. The patients are all of a superior class and had some 1000 pounds with them in their gig, which was run away with and upset, beyond Capheaton, while the men were fighting. One of the Smugglers was very submissive before the Magistrate, the other not so. The Excisemen were quite unarmed when they attempted to seize the Whisky – 4 pistols which they had in their gig, were all uncharged.

I have pleasure to remain
Your affectionate Son
Edward Spencer Trevelyan

A second letter dated June 14th 1830 read as follows:

My Dear Mother

Mr Evans has some awkward symptoms, indicative, but not decidedly, of concussion. Mr Cooper is better. Mr Griffiths son and daughter arrived here early morning, having left Alnwick, last night, as soon as they heard of the business. They were followed by Mr. Evans's wife and son, and 3 or 4 male friends in post-chaises. They were of course much affected by the wretched appearance of their friends' countenances. Mr G's face is entirely covered in plaister. Except the eyes. Miss G is pretty and I have reason to think one of the male friends is her sweetheart. I showed the gardens to the whole party, who have returned to Alnwick excepting Mr G's son and daughter and Mrs Evans, who intend staying at Cambo till their friends are out of danger. I have asked

> Wallington, June 12th Sunday. 1830
> Newcastle on Tyne —
>
> My dear Mother,
> I have had a very busy time of it for the last 28 hours. About 1 o'cl. yesterday, a man rode up to the front door, & rang the bell — He was covered with blood & mud, & could not keep his legs, when he dismounted — I got him washed; & as soon as he could speak, I learnt that he was one of 3 persons connected with the Excise, who had been engaged with 2 Irish Smugglers, a short way south of Little Harle Guide Post, & that he had left his 2 companions lying dead or nearly so, on the road — I immediately sent Creighton & his man to assist them, & they were brought here, in a dreadful state. The heads of all three were almost entire wounds from bludgeon, the skull bared in many places: one of them, M'. Griffiths

8. Edward's handwritten letter June 12th, 1830.

the ladies to Tea this Evening. They all appear highly respectable. Sir J.S. will, I expect, examine the witnesses to-morrow, and the wounded men also : he seems likely to make a bungling job of it. My lions today seemed much pleased with the gardens etc. The trees excited many comparisons to the disadvantage of the Duke's grounds at Alnwick. I cannot speak to highly of the skill and attention Isaac Milburn has shewn in the case of these men. He is so skilful in surgical operations and knows so much of medicine. I don't know what we would have done without him. Mr Hawdon I never saw before, but, despite reports to his disadvantage, I conceived a favourable opinion of him, from the skilful and workman-like manner in which he operated. Alnwick was quite in a ferment till it was known that the men were taken. One of them in answer to Charlton, who is working here, said " The fight lasted 20 minutes, but, my word, there was sharp giving and taking!"

The Smugglers called at *Shaftoe Westhouse*, as they were running away, and got the blood washed off their faces and heads: the occupier will not own to this. Isaac, during the chase searched the house of one Lynn near Shaftoe, who keeps a whisky shop.

Edward then ends his letter describing the garden - a large show of grapes and plums – the Greenhouses in great beauty – It is the 1st time I have been through the Gardens this year.

A further letter below mentioning the smugglers was also documented by Frank Graham, a well-known 20th century north-east author, who mentions a published pamphlet by an unknown author containing these letters entitled "Correspondence Smugglers and Poachers 1830-33 "- as follows:

Carlisle 16th August 1830
===

Dear Sir,

> *I have pleasure of forwarding you by the direction of Mr Justice Bayley a Reprieve for these two Men ; and will thank you to acknowledge the receipt to me at the Bush Inn by return of Post.*
>
> *I am, Dear Sir.*
>
> *Yours Truly*
>
> *Chris. Jno.Newstead.*
>
> *To the Sheriff of the County of Northumberland, and his Under Sheriff; and to the Gaoler or Keeper of His Majesty's Gaol at Morpeth in and for the said County.*
>
> *Let the execution of Peter O'Hara and William Kennedy who were attainted, at the last Assizes held in and for the County of Northumberland on Wednesday the eleventh day of August instant be respited until his Majesty's pleasure be known respecting them.*

Dated this sixteenth day of August 1830. J.Bayley.

Frank Graham states that nothing is known about the publication of the pamphlet, neither the date nor the publisher. The copy was provided by a Mrs Pauline Dower and Mrs P Jennings. He also goes on to mention that "the letters reveal how unwilling Sir John Swinburne was to have the smugglers arrested and punished. Probably like many others, including members of the aristocracy and the clergy, he turned a blind eye on their work, for which service he would occasionally find a barrel of brandy on his doorstep. Poaching was different. Letters show that here the landowners and farmers were united and active in dealing with them. To all landowners poaching was the greatest crime in the calendar but to some smuggling was not. These brief documents are of great social interest providing much insight into the life at Wallington Hall, and the state of medicine in Northumberland in the first half of the 19th Century"

It looks like Isaac played a significant part detaining the smugglers with the use of firearms and provided a helping hand in assisting the recovery of the three excise men which probably enhanced his reputation by word of mouth throughout the Morpeth and Alnwick areas. The final fate of the smugglers is not certain as they seem to have been given a reprieve from execution but that might have been a temporary one. Death records did not start until 1837 so it's more difficult to check.

Life at Wallington Hall August 1833

A few years after the smuggling incident Maria Jane Trevelyan (age 61) wrote a letter on Tuesday August 20th 1833 to her husband Sir John Trevelyan (age 72) the 5th Baronet and head of the family at this time at Wallington Hall with an update on the comings and goings at the hall and nearby vicinity.

It starts in French "Mon cher Epoux" - (my dear husband) - and mentions the weather, visiting their neighbour a Mr Cookson whose proposed new house which will be "very conspicuous and ornamental to the county" and how the road to Hartburn was so "execrably bad" that she returned by Meldon and Bolam. Fruit grown in the estate gardens and heated glasshouses highlight the luxuries of the wealthy estate owners - "melons are coming well on and our allowance of peaches has seldom exceeded six, oftener less." Fruit is nearly over, currants are finished and only gooseberries left that are netted. "The grapes this year are worthless. Peaches very indifferent, cucumbers frequently bitter. The gardeners are mowing round the house."

There is a fascinating description of a journey from London to Wallington Hall by her daughter also called Maria (age 36) and Noel her five-year old grandson.

> *"They started from Blackwall (by ship from docks in London) last Wednesday at 2 O'clock A:M had a very good passage, though rather rough of the coast of Yorkshire for a day and night, and*

got to Shields (the port at the mouth of the river Tyne) about 8 on Friday morning. Captn. Johnstone was on board. He is going to make observations on the Magnet. Miss Bosanquet was also of the party and Ld (Lord) Decies' carriage, 6 servants, 4 Horses & 6 cages of birds."

Maria describes that she has employed another kitchen maid and will see how she gets on with Mrs Walsh who she supposes is very cross. The new maid cooks well and makes goodish bread, but not as good as Mrs Bonsal.

A Kit. Blackett called last week. He is gone to London to place his boy at Harrow.

"In consequence of the birds in the museum not being properly cased the moths have got amongst them and some of the best destroyed. Those which were left in their original cases remain uninjured. The damage may be estimated at £40.

Maria refers to her son Edward Spencer as Spencer and that his horse a mare died of "violent inflammation on Sunday, a sudden attack" and asks if her husband will give him another. Maria thinks Spencer will be married on the 4th September - the marriage actually took place on the 5th to Catherine Anne Forster. Maria goes on to write "It is thought here a very good match for him. The Belsay family all think well of Catherine, & Mr Redman has known her from a child and considers her very amiable, so I daresay Spencer will have done very well for himself "

"Moor game are exceedingly abundant this year." There is mention of a group of shooters at **Hareshaw** that "bagged 47 brace" and another party including a Mat. Bell killing "25 brace the first day" which will be referring to the start of the red grouse shooting season in August known as the glorious 12th. "A brood of 16 Partridges is in the Garden, &, as usual, one of 13 about the house." There is no specific mention of Isaac in this section of the letter but it is safe to assume that as a senior gamekeeper he would have been involved in the shooting and bird rearing activities. Spencer has only been shooting once.

Poaching

Gamekeepers at this time had the power to order poachers off the land and there were severe penalties. Up to 1816 poachers could be forced to join the army or navy. By 1827 sentences up to 14 years transportation to a British colony or three years hard labour for assaulting gamekeepers or threatening violence were introduced. From 1831 fines, with imprisonment in default of payment, were introduced. Trespass in pursuit of rabbits and game attracted a fine of up to £2 plus costs. In a group of five or more a £5 fine and a period of jail was handed out. The hunting of game on any land without a game certificate might result in a fine of up to £5 plus costs or two months in jail. Poaching would not be entered into lightly without thought of the consequences as these would be huge sums of money and severe penalties for the working class and poor to incur.

Generally across the land a lot of working country folk did not accept the game laws, believing them unfair' and poaching the odd rabbit and salmon was considered acceptable. They placed reliance on the Bible in justifying their poaching activities; animals were created for the benefit and service of all mankind, not just the rich.

Genesis 1:26, King James Bible - published in 1611: "And God said, Let us make man in our image, after our likeness: and let them have dominion over the fish of the sea, and over the fowl of the air, and over the cattle, and over all the earth, and over every creeping thing that creepeth upon the earth." Further reading and an in depth analysis on poaching for those interested is available online in a thesis written by Rosemary Muge. (PR6)

Land owners and farmers held quite different views and Maria Trevelyan lets her husband know that, on a nearby estate at Woodburn owned by the Bells, "they were tired of the damage to crops and loss of sheep carried out by poachers and that they had been very daring this year". Her son Spencer had travelled to Woodburn, approx. 12 miles west of Wallington, to assist with others in an attack on the poachers. The group assembled at Woodburn consisted of 46 on horses and 60 on foot made up of four mounted dragoons, three infantry, 4 policemen, "gentlemen", farmers from the neighbourhood, their watchers (lookouts for poachers) and gamekeepers.

The Wallington contingent arrived at Woodburn at half past eight on Monday evening and returned Wednesday afternoon with an account of the events that took place written up by Maria in her letter :

> "They started at 3 o'clock yesterday morning in two divisions, one consisting of 30 horse headed by Mr Charles Brandling & Sir Thos Haggerstone both magistrates and in which Spencer and his horsemen went, to the Carter near which place a part of poachers had been seen proceeding up the road 18 in number. Upon being pursued they left the hill by the course of a burn which formed a sort of coombe (a small valley), about half way up which they were overtaken, when they formed themselves into a body on a steep bank about 12 or 15 yards above the bed of the burn, and, upon a nearer approach of the attacking party, they presented arms & made use of the most violent threats. After allowing them time to vent their rage, the other party who were armed with pistols and cutlasses, closed with them, and, after a short struggle, the poachers, who did not make use of any violent

or deadly efforts to escape, were all disarmed and captured with their 18 guns & 12 dogs. They were taken to Whitelees bar, & sent off on carts to Morpeth Gaol. The persons who were most active & daring in the attack were those watchers who had been poachers themselves. In going down Harwood an accident occurred by which one of the poachers had his leg broken which was a consequence of his jumping out of the cart in an attempt to escape. A policeman had his shoulder dislocated when his gig was run away". Two other poachers who were handcuffed together also jumped out of the cart, and made for Catcherside plantation, but were soon recaptured.

"The other division, headed by Mat. & Charles Bell, succeeded in taking 4 out of 6 poachers near Greenhaugh. The same day a party of six poachers were seen at Ottercaps & Birkett burn, but the watchers being absent with the other party, they were not interfered with. At the beginning of the (grouse) season a party of poachers 5 in number took possession of a farm house near Hesleyside for the night, but were taken by Mr Charlton, who, having deprived them of their guns, very weakly and foolishly liberated them. The guns were taken to Dixon the steward's house Mantle Hill, whose house the next day was besieged by a large gang demanding the guns, and Mr Dixon, not wishing to outshine his master in valor, restored them. Joe Stott the Harwood watcher behaved very well at the battle of Whitelee.

Spencer has given directions for forts to be built on the most commanding situations on the Wallington moors which will be properly garrisoned and telegraphic communication (probably hand written letters) is to be established with all the surrounding moorland district. Spencer wishes you to appoint him governor of these forts with a salary not exceeding £500 per annum."

Surprisingly given Isaac's contribution to the rounding up of the smugglers, I found it hard to believe he was not part of the search party or mentioned in being involved in treating the injuries suffered by both the policeman and the poachers. It turns out Isaac had other duties taking carts full of game to Morpeth on the Tuesday and Marie Trevelyan mentions him specifically in her letter stating that he had not yet returned by quarter past 11 on the Wednesday evening. Maybe a trip to the market town was a thirsty exercise and involved a few beers at the local hostelries !!

Historical context – A few years after this tale in 1838 Samuel Morse invented the Morse Code.

CHAPTER 3

LEAVING WALLINGTON HALL

Part time practice interest to full-time bonesetter

Isaac is recorded at the age or 45 in the 1841 census, still working as a gamekeeper living at the Dovecote Wallington with his wife Elizabeth 40 and his sons William 15, Robert 5 and mother-in-law Jane Thornton age 90. His daughter Jane 16 was now working as a drape maker's apprentice in Newgate St, Morpeth.

Broken horse comes home

Early in 1846 one of the horses on the Wallington estate fell, broke its leg and Isaac was ordered by Spencer Trevelyan to have it shot and destroyed. Given what we know so far this would probably have been a straightforward task for Isaac. However it would appear that this was not the case and was against Isaac's principles. Interestingly his aim with the horse was to cure not to destroy. Isaac obviously thought he had the knowledge to fix the break, take a risky gamble and go against his master's instructions. So, unknown to Spencer Trevelyan, he repaired the damaged limb and soon had the horse fit and well, whereupon he took it to a market, most likely at Morpeth, to be sold at auction. By coincidence, Trevelyan also attended the auction and liked the look of the horse as it reminded him of the one he had lost so he made the purchase.

On arriving back at Wallington Hall the horse walked straight into its own stall!!

Spencer Trevelyn was very angry, no doubt a bit embarrassed and probably felt let down by Isaac. Knowing of Isaac's bone setting activities, with sufferers now coming from far and near to be cured of their injuries, he instructed Mr Gow the estates land agent to write him a letter saying "he would have to make his choice between being head gamekeeper or bone-setter for the county" – one or the other. Mr Gow is described by Edward Keith as the most important power behind the scenes at Wallington Hall for half a century during the life of four baronet owners. He was an able, far-seeing man and looked after the business between the owners and the estates farm tenants. Dealing with an incident like the horse on behalf of Spencer Trevelyan would therefore be straightforward for a man of his standing and save Trevelyan any further conflict.

Isaac made a relatively quick but nevertheless important decision to quit his job at Wallington Hall and was resolved to make bone-setting his long-term aim in his life.

These were uncertain and tough times for the working class in rural settings. There were many desperately poor people roaming the countryside looking for work and a place to live. Farmers renting farms from wealthy landowners would provide some employment but they relied heavily on good weather for crops and fair prices for corn and livestock in order that their business might survive. Those seeking work on farms would attend "hirings" at Morpeth and other market towns on set days of the year.

According to a well-respected local Throphill farmer called William Brewis, who kept diaries, (PR7) at this time there were many farms up for let as the farmers were struggling to make ends meet. Brewis was also a High Constable of Morpeth and mentions meeting Isaac for dinner on the 23rd March 1846 at a nearby farm called Thropton.

Given this background Isaac must have felt very confident and undaunted as his first step was to continue working as a gamekeeper for an unknown but brief period at Brinkburn, an estate approximately 13 miles north east of Wallington Hall, owned at the time by Cadogan Hodgson. Subsequently he set up as an innkeeper at the Bird in Bush pub in Elsdon where he worked for a short while or so to continue his bone setting practice. Set beside a beautiful village green the pub still retains a lot of original features including a very small window large enough to pass a glass of beer through to any visiting drovers who were not allowed inside !!

This early combination of a pub and bone setting was to become a significant business model for his future bone setting career. However, on some occasions as the following case describes, Isaac would travel to see a patient if their medical condition prevented them from travelling.

Wagon way man

Amongst other local cases deserving of record is that of a man, who having got off the road at night between Shilbottle and Alnwick, wandered on to the old wagon way and fell over into the coal depot. He was picked up the next morning a cripple, and for three weeks could only move with the help of crutches. Medical skill seemed of no avail. He was persuaded to place himself in Isaac's hands, who came from Elsdon, to perform the operation. After placing the lame foot in hot water for some time, he was able to force the misplaced tendons into their proper position, and the man found that for the first time since his accident he was able to place his foot to the ground.

> *"Now my man"* said Isaac
> *"I'll hav to see thee walking before I gan"*

The man insisted he could not go without his crutches, but Isaac was equally insistent that he should, and the result was that the man, after a few trials, was able to walk across the room with perfect ease.

The early part of 1846 was certainly a year of change and disruption for the Milburn family as documents also describe Isaac working at one of the village inns in Longframlington with his family. He managed this establishment for a number of years, where he continued to practise his 'humane art' and was looked upon as being almost supernatural. There were seven inns in or near to Longframlington on a map of 1866 where Isaac might have resided, namely The Horse and Jockey, New Inn, Grand B Inn, Queens Head Inn, Rimside Moor House Inn/Swinburne Arms (near Moor House farm), The Anglers Arms and Besom Inn – a somewhat thirsty area. I suspect Isaac worked at the Rimside Moor House Inn which was owned by John and Elizabeth Wardle as there is a Wardle connection described a little bit further on, and records show that Isaac is not named as proprietor in any of the other inns.

Isaac's first press advert that I have found online appears in 1846 as follows –

ISAAC MILBURN Bonesetter & VETERINARY SURGEON

Begs to inform his friends and the public that he will attend every alternate Tuesday (commencing 16th May) at the house of Robert Strappen, Bluebell Inn, Clayport, Alnwick.

NB Horses stifles and slipped shoulders adjusted. Framlington May 14th 1846.

As well as expanding his work area to cover Alnwick and surrounding places he is also treating animals as well. I have only found a few other examples of his work with animals but it seems that he was equally ready to do what he could for suffering domestic pets as he would for their owners.

Church cat

In a Presbyterian manse in north Northumberland there lived a favourite cat, which, in one of her night time rambles, had the misfortune to get one of her legs so badly injured as to be of no service. She lay on the hearthrug disconsolate and spiritless or hirpled about painfully on three feet, an object of pity to all concerned. As a rule a cat is its own best doctor when its sufferings arise from a flesh wound developing into a suppurating sore. But here was a purely surgical case, beyond pussy's reach. Anyone who has assisted at a surgical operation on a cat, as did the writer (of Isaacs biography) once in cutting a fish-hook out of a Tom's lip, would be in no hurry to try attempt a second. The animal's whole body became surcharged, as it were, with nerve power, and his twistings and writhings grew so intense that only those who witnessed them could realise the almost supernatural power displayed. With a woman's quick wit and rapid decision, the maid at the manse determined to consult with Isaac upon the state of Tabby's leg. Carrying her off she submitted her charge to Isaac's inspection. The bonesetter seemed to possess a strange power of allaying the cats' natural aversion to a stranger, and without ever running the risk of a scratch or attempted flight he set a dislocated joint, and returned the cat with the free use of her leg, and would take no fee for his services.

His area of practice continued to expand, and another similar advert appears on the 10th July in the same year in the Newcastle Courant:

ISAAC MILBURN Bonesetter

Begs to inform his friends and the public that he will attend every alternate Tuesday (commencing on the 21st July) at the house of Mr Wm Hall, Goat Inn, Cloth Market, Newcastle and trusts unremitting attention to his profession to merit their support. Longframlington May 14 1846.

The Goat Inn is an interesting establishment and appears to have been of a type similar to our present micro-breweries. The owner William Hall ran a brewery attached to the inn on the ground floor producing ten half-barrels at each brewing - source Brian Bennison. (PR8)

Isaac was a plain, blunt man, who did not hesitate to swear at a feint hearted patient who might moan over his sufferings and seemed inclined to start crying in prospect of the planned treatment. But to women he could be as gentle and tender as if he had in him nothing but the "milk of human kindness". With boys he was so familiar and jocular that he disarmed all fear and made them forget that they were in the hands of a man who, if he was to do them any good at all, would have to inflict a degree of pain. Dislocated joints had their terror spirited away by the winning words and tact which the experienced man knew when and how to employ.

A simple example of his down to earth character, without any airs and graces, is highlighted by the fact that he always wanted to be called Isaac and not the formal "Mr Milburn"

An extract from Isaac's biography printed by the Newcastle Courant in 1879 explains as follows:

> *Isaac – and here let the sticklers for precise etiquette understand that the apparent familiar use of the Christian name arises from no disrespect to the bearer of it, but solely from deference to the frank, manly bluntness which makes him prefer the plain "Isaac" to the stiffer and more formal "Mister" – he is emphatically, and by his oft repeated declaration,*
>
> *"Isaac" not "Mister"*
>
> *- a distinction with a difference, which to the wise will afford no little insight into his character.*

A lot of the undated cases which follow were written about in newspaper articles and are without any names other than in some cases their initials to preserve their identity as presumably no permission had been given.

Tyneside man

A young man belonging to one of the Tyneside towns sustained an injury to his knee by what at the time was thought to be a straightforward fall. After some delay surgical advice was taken and many measures were prescribed to alleviate the pain but with no success. Weeks of constant suffering and sleeplessness began to tell upon the patient's health which ultimately gave way to such an extent that his case became one rather for the physician than the surgeon. To his family and their doctor it became more and more evident day by day that the young man was suffering from consumption - an old and once common term for wasting away of the body, particularly from pulmonary tuberculosis (TB). The initial cause being deemed to be the fall, the state of his knee which resulted in lameness. He was ordered to travel inland for a change of air and so ended up in Morpeth where he had to place himself under the care of a local doctor that also believed in the consumption diagnosis. His landlady having heard the history of his ailments persuaded him to consult Isaac who found him to be suffering from a dislocation. Having given him certain oils to rub the part he was able at his next visit to replace the joint and to his doctor's great surprise when next he went to visit him the young man was walking outside the house with the aid of only a stick instead of moving about on two crutches an apparently dying man.

"Hows this come about?" was the doctors first words,

"Oh I've been to see Isaac" said the young man.

"Damn Isaac" said the learned doctor, who turned on his heel and abruptly walked away.

Here we have an example of how doctors and physicians of the time may possibly have been lacking in training, experience and medical knowledge which probably created a resentment to unregulated practitioners of "bone-setting" like Isaac. Nowadays I guess resetting a dislocation by well-trained physicians is straightforward but back in the 19th century it would seem this would have led to immeasurable suffering for the working man and woman.

A somewhat difficult and demanding year for Isaac as his mother Elizabeth (nee Thornton) died at Thornhill in 1846.

Mrs A Luke from Hedley-on-the-Hill, Isaac's great granddaughter, commented in the 1960s that she was in the possession of a beautiful silver service tea service, which was given to Isaac by the people of Longframlington. It is understood that a subscription was instigated by a Mrs Elizabeth Wardle, known as "Betty Wardle" who was the grateful owner of the once famed bakery, the "Moor House". The teapot, sugar basin and cream server were presented to him at the bakery and inscribed on the teapot are the words 'To Mr. Isaac Milburn, of Framlington, by a few friends, as a Testimonial of their regard for his talent and general humane conduct towards relieving his fellow creatures – 1847'

There does not appear to be any records of a bakery at Moor House but there was certainly a successful inn called the Swinburne Arms or more commonly known as the Rimside Moor House Inn on the main drover's road from Scotland to Morpeth run by Elizabeth Wardle a few miles north of Longframlington. This is now a private house but there are tales of ghosts, murders and highwaymen in this relatively isolated area and at one time a gibbet stood opposite the inn.

As Isaac reached the age of 55 the 1851 census states the family are all living in the same household in Longframlington with his wife Elizabeth, daughter Jane, 26, and the two sons William, 24, and Robert, 15. His daughter Jane's marriage at "Framlington" is announced in the Newcastle Guardian and Mercury on the 1st October 1854 to Mr. W. Leighton of Thirsleyhaugh only daughter of Isaac Milburn bonesetter.

Another advert in 1854 detailed below shows that he has changed his "pub surgery" in Alnwick to that of the Nags Head.

> ISAAC MILBURN,
> BONE SETTER AND VETERINARY SURGEON,
> BEGS to inform his friends and the public that he will attend every alternate Saturday (commencing on the 27th of May) at the house of Mr Dunn, Nag Head Inn, Fenkle-street, Alnwick; and trusts, by unremitting attention to his profession, to merit their support, which he has most thankfully received.
> Framlington, May 15, 1854.

9. 19th May, 1854 Newcastle Courant Advert.

Sadly his wife Elizabeth's death is in the Alnwick Mercury newspaper a few years later on November 17th 1857 at Longframlington, aged 57 much respected wife of Isaac Milburn bonesetter.

An advert in the Alnwick Mercury on Friday 1st January 1858 is as follows:

Isaac Milburn begs to announce to his friends and the public in general that he has removed from Framlington to Dunsheugh in the parish of Longhoughton and will attend at Alnwick Morpeth and other places upon the same days as he has formerly done, where every attention and punctuality may be relied upon. Dunsheugh Jan 1st 1858.

By the next census in 1861 Isaac is living on his own at Dunsheugh, a small farmstead beside Ratcheugh Observatory a few miles to the east of Alnwick.

Regular adverts continue in the Alnwick Mercury June 1860, 2nd Feb 1863 and on the 1st April 1864 as follows:

Isaac Milburn Bonesetter Dunsheugh will be at Misses Dunn's Nags Head Inn Alnwick every Saturday and at the Black Bull Inn Morpeth on Wednesday 13th and every alternative Wednesday.

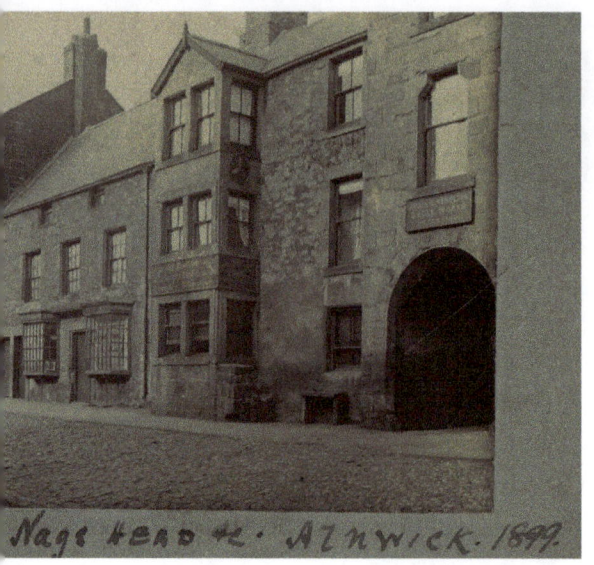
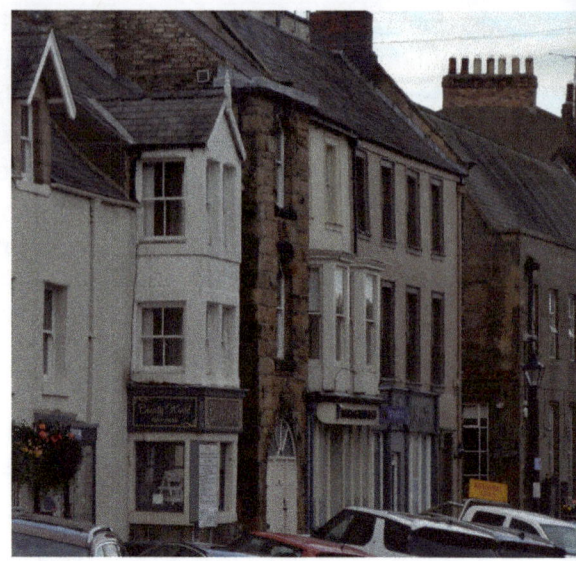

10a / 10b. The Nags Head Inn past and present on Fenkle Street Alnwick.

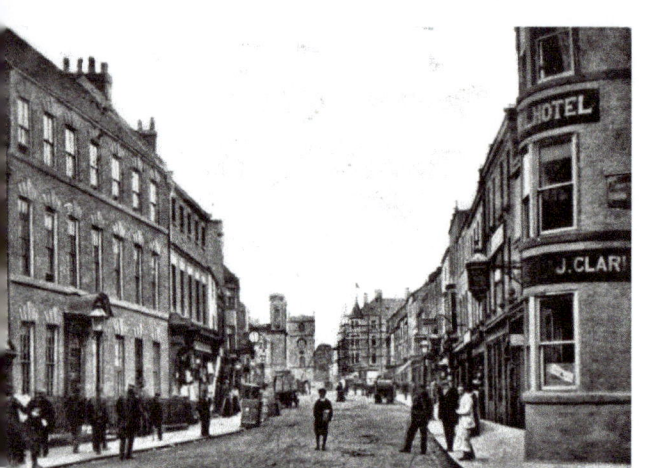
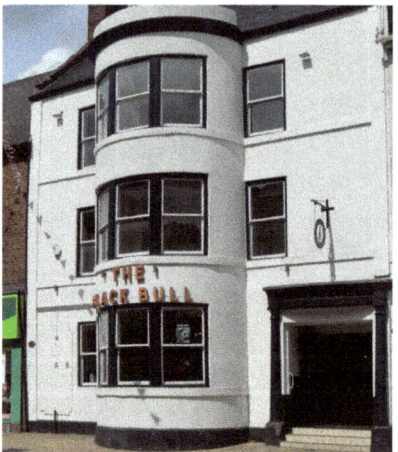

11a / 11b. The Black Bull Hotel, Morpeth, past and present.

A few years later the Morpeth Herald announced Isaac's second marriage at Rennington church on the 24th October 1863 by the Rev W.L.J. Cooley. Mr Isaac Milburn the celebrated bonesetter of Dunsheugh to Miss Margaret Whittle of Low Hocket near Alnwick.

Isaac was 68 and Elizabeth was 56.

On June 1st 1863 Isaac is mentioned in "John Blacks Diary" (PR9) an account of when he was asked to attend an accident at his farm, where he lived, called Ford Westfield, a few miles to the south of Ford in north Northumberland. John Black also managed Hay farm, and farms at Kimmerston,

Heatherslaw and its mill. His brother George was responsible for Ford Forge and the spadework's at Spittal. My thanks to David Lockie, who took possession of the diary and gave a number of talks on the contents, and his wife Mary who sent me the diary entry below.

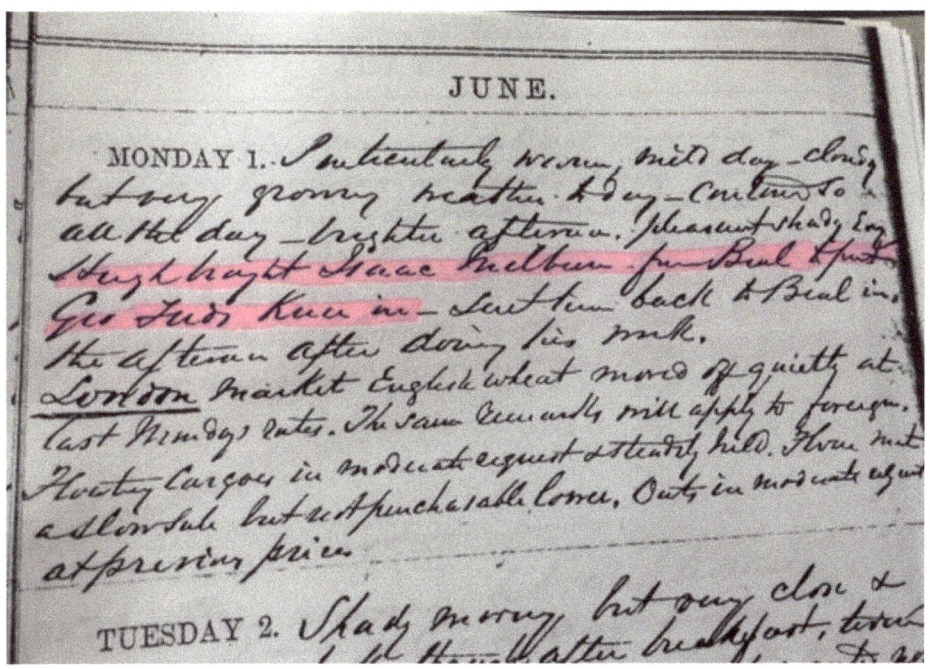

The diary records that it was a "particularly warm mild day- cloudy but very growing weather - continued so all day - brighter afternoon, pleasant shady". Isaac was brought, no doubt by horse drawn transport, the 10 miles from Beal by Hugh to put back in the knee of George Ford who was presumably a farm worker. Isaac most likely travelled up by train to Beal railway station or may have been staying in the area at this time before his wedding. We know from the 1861 Census records that his son William was living at nearby East Kyloe cottages and working as an agricultural labourer which is close to Beal.

Isaac moved from Dunsheugh and set up home with his new wife at Drive Cottage at some point about this time. Drive Cottage is a short distance south of Longbank Farm which is south of Longhoughton and was near the site of an old tile works.

There is a record in Alnwick Castle Archives for 1865 of Isaac renting land in the form of a garden from the Duke of Northumberland's Estate at Longhougton for an annual rent of £3 (ACA/Agmt/A3268). It was beside the tile works which were part of Long Bank Farm. According to a survey

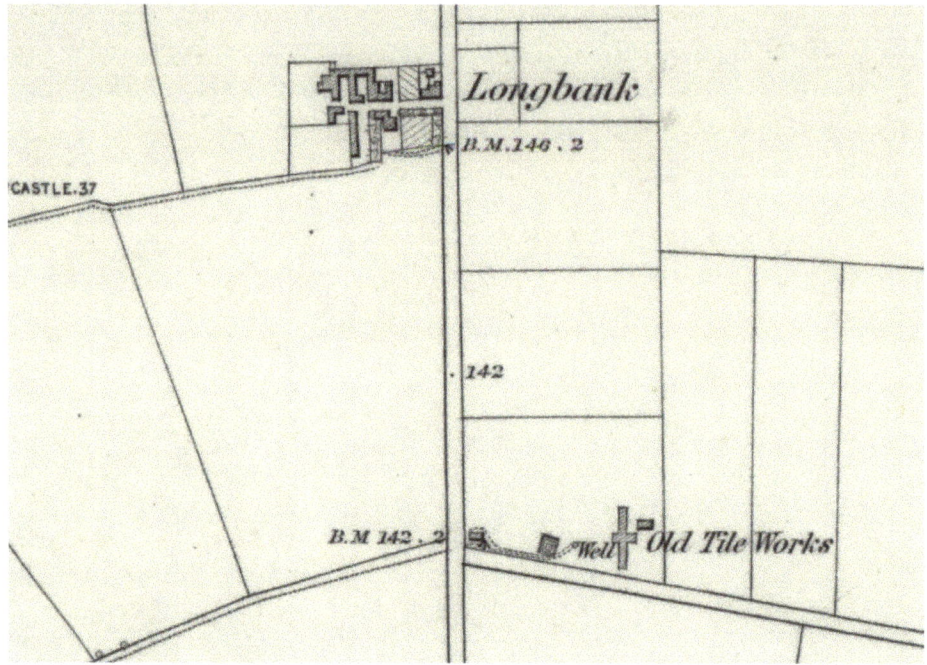

12. Drive Cottage map.

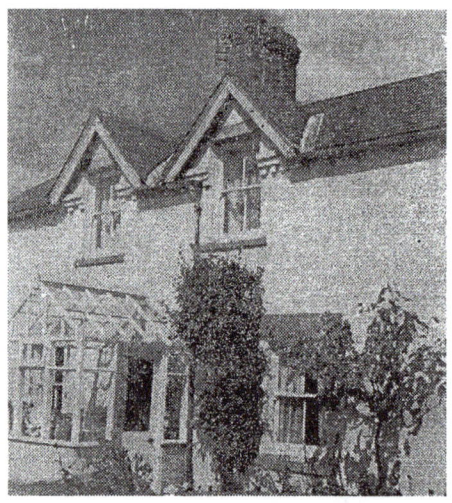

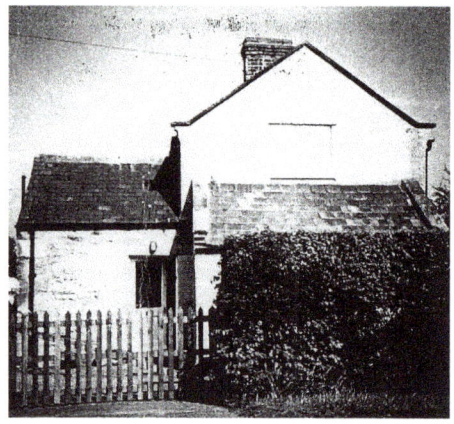

13, above / 14, left. Drive Cottage - Longhoughton in the 1960s.

in 1850 Isaac's cottage is described as being situated at Longhoughton Tilery in the Township of LongHoughton. The tilery was in the occupation of Hall and Creighton as Tilery Lessees.

This was a time of great industrial progress with the East coast railway opening between Newcastle and Tweedmouth in 1847 and the Royal Border Bridge completing the link to Berwick upon Tweed in 1850 when it was opened by Queen Victoria. Isaac made full use of this new, and what we can only imagine must have appeared to be incredibly faster form of transport compared to horse and carriage, travelling by train from nearby Longhoughton station to places such as Tweedmouth, Morpeth and Newcastle on market days to carry out his bone setting profession. These would certainly be at their busiest on market days with people from the countryside and nearby villages travelling in to buy and sell goods. The railway may possibly have been one of his reasons for his move to Longhoughton, with its own station and easier connections to his patients. By 1863 three passenger trains left Longhoughton station on weekdays for Morpeth and Newcastle, at 7.25am, 1.00pm and 6.35pm.

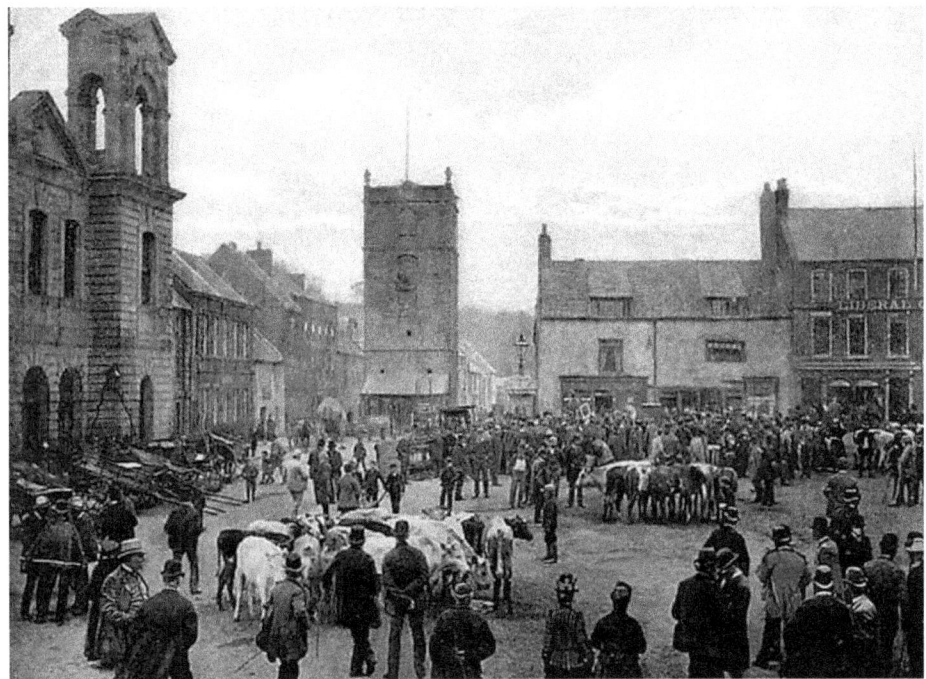

15. Morpeth market late 1800s

Station baby

It is mentioned by Mary Kipling that "many miners had reason to be grateful to Isaac, as many an injured limb was repaired by him on the station platform. On one occasion a woman greatly distressed and carrying an infant, begged him to attend her baby. He took the crying child into his arms and in seconds, he repaired the dislocation of the shoulder, just before the train began to move out of the station. The overjoyed mother took her baby from him and her grateful thanks followed him until the train moved out of sight, from the station"

Continued technological advances meant that the Royal Mail was now leaving London at 9 o'clock in the evening and taking 12 hours between London and Newcastle whereas previously it had taken two days. Steam ships were departing from Liverpool to cross the Atlantic to New York with a journey time between 12 and 14 days.

CHAPTER 4
ISAAC'S CASEBOOK

And so to more of Isaac's cases from various newspaper accounts.

Young River Wear Lady

This case from the Newcastle Courant article was "that of a young lady, tall, handsome, beautiful, who had the misfortune a few winters ago to slip on an icy pavement in one of the towns on the banks of the River Wear, and thus severely spraining her foot and ankle. Her position in life enabled her to command the best surgical skill in the north of England, and everything was done to mitigate the severity of the pain, and at the same time keep up her general health. The recovery of the foot would be a matter of time, and for once the doctors were right. The time – weary long months – proved an absolute certainty, but the recovery of the use of the foot came not. Dreading the prospect of being a cripple for life, she at last determined to abandon her professional advisers, and see what the much vaunted but much dreaded and half suspected Isaac could do for her. Unable to touch the ground with her foot, she was conveyed to lodgings within reach of one of the Northumbrian towns regularly visited by Isaac. At his first examination he found the flesh and ligaments of the foot so much swollen and stiffened that nothing definite could be ascertained. Giving directions how to subdue the swelling and relax the muscles was all that could be done on that occasion. Next week he was able, from the more pliable state of the foot, to find that at least one small bone had been dislocated and to suspect that there were others in the same condition. The joint having been replaced the sufferer was rejoiced to find that she could at least let her foot touch the floor, and thus encouraged she implicitly followed Isaac's directions. Another visit completed the operation and in less than a week she was able to take daily exercise on the highway, with the aid of a staff and supporting arm of a friend. For some weeks she continued to have it re-examined and re-bandaged by the experienced hands of the old man. Her gratitude to him was unbounded and she often declared that she would pray for him while he lived, and felt sure that, if any man would go to heaven at last it would be Isaac Milburn, bonesetter and gentleman in the highest sense of the word.

Public servant and wife

There are many examples of his knowledge and aptness both to diagnose and repair an injury to sinews and tendons which is tissue that unites muscle to the bone. A public servant, who came into almost daily contact with him while travelling to and from on his errands of mercy, but who had regarded him as only a sort of quack, fell lame in one of his feet, and so continued for some time. Taking advantage of Isaac's casual presence one day at his place of business he asked him to look at his foot. In less time than it takes to tell the story, a tendon which had got thrown out of position, was replaced, and bandaged, and in a day or two the pain and lameness were both gone. The same man's wife suffered at one time from severe pain in her right arm, which gradually became so weak that she was glad to carry it about in a sling. After much persuasion she consented to have it examined by Isaac, who not only readjusted an injured sinew but told her that it had been produced by over-exertion at the washing tub – a fact which she knew and admitted.

Soldier

In his long and varied experience many remarkable cases passed through Isaac's hands' but perhaps there is not one better than a man known as "T.T". a soldier, who served his country during the Indian mutiny 1857 – a major rebellion and unsuccessful uprising in India against the rule of the British East India Company, which functioned as a sovereign power on behalf of the British Crown. In one of the battles in which the soldier was engaged he was shot in the breast, the bullet passing through this body and escaping just behind his shoulder. He recovered from his wound, but with an arm that hung powerless by his side. The regimental surgeons certified him as unfit for further service, and he was accordingly discharged with the usual pension. Returning to his home in Northumberland, he went about as "a broken soldier" with no prospect but to eke out, what might be a long life, on the slender bounty granted by his country. His friends, however, took heart of grace, and induced him, notwithstanding the opinion of the army doctors as to his permanent disablement, to submit his arm and shoulder to the inspection of Isaac. To the astonishment and surprise of all, Isaac declared that the blow of the bullet had put his shoulder out, and ultimately proved the truth of his discovery by putting it in, and restoring to the pensioned soldier the use of his arm, which for many long years after took its fair share with the other in the heavy lifts demanded of a mason's labourer.

If you wish to gain an insight into the degree of pain associated with a dislocated shoulder and how a modern-day hospital will tackle the problem then take a look at the following You Tube link.

https://www.youtube.com/watch?v=HzROgg-HWPk

The Doctor

The following story was told to Mary Kipling.

> Isaac with his straightforward personality had little time for those that who doubted his ability or tried to take a rise out of him.
>
> A very young doctor, who was sceptical of Isaac's ability, decided to pay him a visit, complaining of pain in his shoulder. He arrived with his arm in a sling, saying his shoulder must be out of joint. Being very perceptive, Isaac soon 'caught on' and giving the offending joint a quick twist, said,
>
> "Well young man, your shoulder wasn't out when you came in, but it is now, and you can get who you like to put it back in"

Windy Gyle – boy and Wooler child

It is acknowledged and folly that none of Isaac's cases turned out badly. The writer of the Courant article met with a little boy at the foot of Windy Gyle – roughly halfway between Rothbury and Jedburgh as the crow flies, in the heart of the Cheviots, whose dislocated elbow had been set by Isaac, but very much needed to be set again. It hung misshapen and slightly shrivelled by his side, and the young lad was unable either to put on or take off his cap with it. The parents, however, did not blame Isaac. They were satisfied he had done his work well; but blamed themselves for having done justice neither to him nor their boy by removing the bandage too soon.

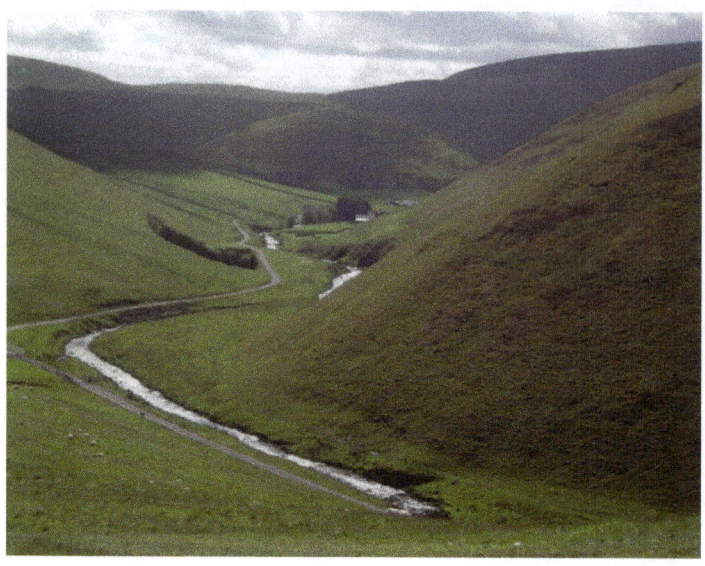

16. Photo of Windy Gyle with credit and permission to use from Shepherds Walks.

This case highlights that suffering patients were prepared to travel great distances to visit Isaac at either of his preferred Alnwick or Morpeth pub surgeries. Having never heard of Windy Gyle, I discovered that it is a hill some 1963 feet/693 metres in height and I set about to find out its whereabouts. It lies close to the England/Scotland border. There are a number of remote properties on the eastern side of Windy Gyle, namely Trows, Rowhope and Windyhaugh – all of which are still quite isolated and windswept sheep farming locations some 28 miles distance west from Alnwick.

So it would have been no mean feat to travel this distance in the mid 1800s – possibly by horse and cart, in pain, initially on a long winding, bumpy farm track through the Coquet Valley to Alwinton and onto Alnwick. There was unfortunately no railway connection in those days as the line between Whittingham and Alnwick did not open until 1887.

Wooler Bairn

A similar example of a patient's keenness and maybe desperation to travel great lengths, in this case about 18 miles by foot, was when a poor woman and child came to the Nags Head in Alnwick about 1880. She had trudged by foot from the neighbourhood of Wooler carrying her maimed offspring in her arms. As soon as she entered Isaac's presence he addressed her in his usual blunt manner as follows:

"where did ye come frae?"

"from Wooler" she replied;

"and what's the matter wi ya"

"oh its no me, it's the bairn who has been lame for three weeks, and the doctors have worked on him all that time, but he is no better".

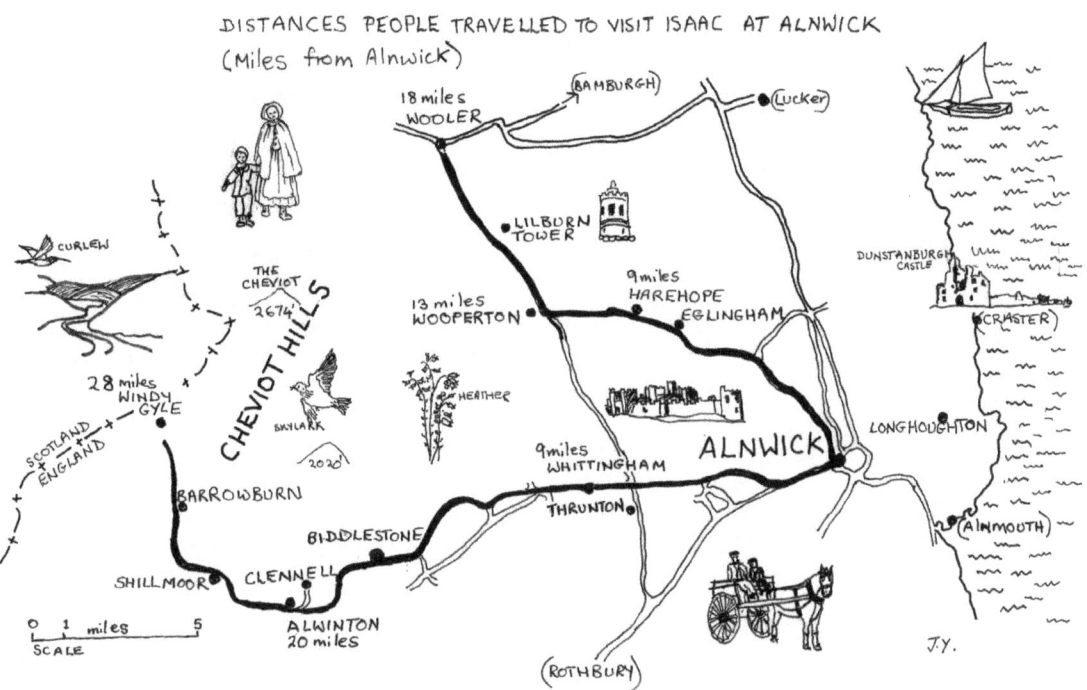

17. Windy Gyle to Alnwick 28 miles. Wooler to Alnwick 18 miles.

Isaac at once took hold of the child's arm and with one twist of his skilful hand the arm was right in an instant. The poor woman was delighted to see her child so soon restored; and at once asked what it was to pay, at the same time adding that she had very little money.

"Well how much hav ye?"

"Only eighteen pence" said the woman, at the same time producing it as a fee.

"How dye ye expect to git hyem again" said the bonesetter.

"Why I will have to walk "

"Walk! the dammed, ye canna walk; keep your money, and here's half a crown, and jist gan and git a ride home with the carrier"

It would appear Isaac had genuine sympathy for hard working people. He made it his practice to give them the benefit of his skill at moderate charges, and was generous to a degree in waiving the normal fee in all cases of extreme and undoubted hardship.

The quantity of cases during Isaac's life show clearly he was a public benefactor. The number he has rescued from what might have been life-long lameness is difficult to calculate and when it is taken into account the families that were saved from hardship which might have seen semi- starvation or the workhouse, the magnitude of his services assumes surprising proportion.

Coal Miners

Those who witnessed the surgery scenes at the Nag's Head Inn at Alnwick, the Black Bull Inn, Morpeth, and noted the numbers of patients queuing to see Isaac, spoke of his work as something wonderful. His average number of cases at Alnwick was nine or ten each week and at Morpeth in the midst of the pit district, where accidents of all kinds were frequent, he often had as many as twenty-five patients through his hands. Many injured coal miners from the pit villages of Blyth and Ashington would arrive at the Morpeth station by railway or other means, injured and lame from frequent mining accidents. Credible witnesses affirm that persons who were carried in, or who with difficulty made their own way in on crutches, were often seen walking out without assistance, or merely the support of a staff.

Historical context – 1876 Alexander Graham Bell invented the telephone. 1878 Joseph Swan a British scientist demonstrated the first electric light with a similar discovery in America by Thomas Edison a few months later. 1881 the first public electricity supply was commenced in Godalming Surrey.

CHAPTER 5

A ROYAL APPOINTMENT, GUNPOWDER, TREASON AND PLOT

Firstly can I say that the gunpowder tale has absolutely nothing to do with Isaac's encounters with royalty. I have just grouped them together to gain attention and show the extreme and diverse characteristics of the man!

John Rowantree's article in the Northumberland Gazette November 1967 (PR10) states that "Isaac was a great friend of the Duke of Northumberland, who was in the habit of calling at Isaac's cottage while travelling on horseback along the "Dukes ride" from Alnwick Castle to the sea coast. It was the Duke who is believed to have arranged for Isaac to treat two of the Royal princesses on separate occasions."

Over many decades his reputation and recommendations from satisfied clients are understood to

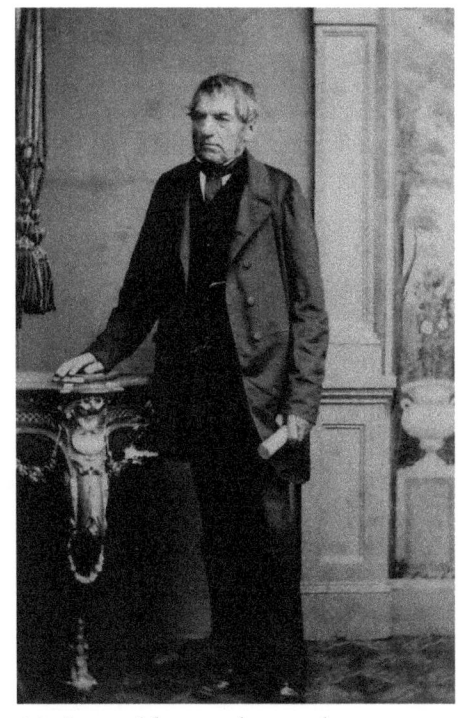

18. Isaac (date unknown).

have resulted in Isaac treating members of the Royal family on a number of occasions in his own characteristic style. I have taken the position that the Royal tales are true although his testimonial and obituary at the time do not mention the Royal names specifically and my guess is that this was because of secrecy and patient confidentiality. I leave it to the reader to make up their own mind.

The following article was written by Mary Kipling in 1967.

Royal Command

The episode concerning Queen Victoria happened when he lived at Drive Cottage, Longhoughton, with his second wife Margaret Whittle. Princess Beatrice, the Queen's young daughter, had received an injury to her hip and in spite of all the skill of the best doctors obtainable, she remained helpless and in great pain.

By this time, Isaac's fame had spread far and wide and the Queen, having heard of his skill as a bonesetter, commanded him to go to the Palace. (I was loaned a photograph of him, holding in his hand the Royal Command).

An 84 year old gentleman, residing at Tosson Towers, Rothbury, and who has since passed on, told me that his father and grandfather knew Isaac very well. He recounted to me in detail, a description of Isaac's arrival at the London station in answer to the Royal Command.

He had been informed that he would be met on arrival at the station. Stepping from the train, he threw up his hands and called out,

"*I am Isaac Milburn, anyone here for me?*".

A gentleman in uniform stepped forward says, "*This way sir*",

and led Isaac to a waiting carriage and pair. The old gentleman continued: "Isaac thought the carriage looked a very shabby one, not quite what he had expected so declined the lift, saying in his Northumberland dialect":

"*A walk in Northumberland, 'a can wa'alk here,*" so he set off to the Palace. On his arrival, he was conducted to the bed-chamber where the Princess lay, in great pain, the Queen sitting very distressed at the foot of the bed.

The room seemed full of eminent gentlemen, doctors, I was told, who no doubt, hoped, to watch Isaac at work.

He was too far north to be caught out like that, so requested that they leave the room, as he preferred to work alone.

He could be very gentle with women and children and after examining the Princess, and diagnosing the trouble, he put the injured joint back into place and turning to the Queen said,

"*What this canny bairn must have suffered but she will be alright now*".

Taking the Princess by the hand, he helped her to her feet. The Queen was overjoyed and with tears raining down her cheeks, she took off her gold watch and chain and gave it to Isaac as a memento.

It was a very proud Isaac who returned to Drive Cottage where his wife was waiting for him, sitting in her chair by the fireside, wearing a black dress and on her head a little white mutch.

Throwing the watch into her lap, he said:

"*There what do you think of that, the Queen's watch*".

He was very proud of it and was never parted from it until his dying day. Some of the people Mary talked to thought it must have been buried with him. However, in 1971, Mary received a letter from a lady in Hexham, great great granddaughter of Isaac, who said it had been in their home, until the home was broken up.

A similar account is also detailed in the Newcastle Courant biography which I believe is the same tale.

Isaac's services have been called into requisition by the nobility and gentry, and he has been summoned on special occasions to travel long distances to attend distinguished patients. Once he was taken up to London to advise on the case of a young lady whose injury had baffled the skill of the first Metropolitan surgeons. On his arrival he found the room occupied not only by her relatives and attendants, but by several gentlemen whose business there he had no difficulty in guessing, but whose presence he neither wanted nor relished. Turning to the patient's father, he asked who these gentlemen were. On being informed that they were the surgeons who had been attending her, he positively refused to even examine the injured limb till they retired. They did so, when he addressed himself to his work and soon announced the nature of the mischief. The father asked if he could do anything for her.

"*Yes*" said Isaac.

"*How long will it be before you can perform the operation*" queried the anxious parent.

For reply, he was told that the time could not be precisely fixed, as it would take him a while to make some preliminary preparations. Ignoring

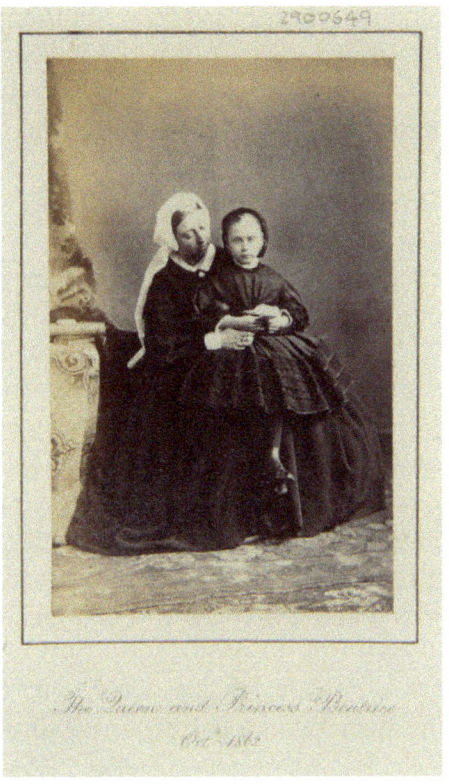

19. Queen Victoria holding Princess Beatrice affectionately called "Baby" in 1862.

alike the father and the adjoining roomful of skilled professors, Isaac proceeded with the duty before him and in twenty minutes he had the limb set, while those around only thought he was getting ready to begin. When informed of the fact the father was almost irate at his not having been told beforehand when the final act was to be done. Isaac was convinced that the design was to summon the surgeons into the room to see it performed; but was "too far north" to be caught in that way, and scrupled not to chuckle over their manifest disappointment, which even the joy at the restoration of the young lady, was not sufficient to make them conceal.

If this is the Princess Beatrice tale then the father would have been Prince Albert who died in 1861. This therefore does not match up exactly with the previous account of Victoria's watch being given to Isaac's second wife as they were married in 1864. One or both of the accounts could have incorrect details or have been deliberately written to hide the true facts to throw people off the scent but still give a sense of importance to his work. It is therefore quite difficult to work out exactly which tale to believe and which facts are correct.

A second Royal encounter, also described by Mary Kipling, occurred after the Buckingham Palace visit with what is thought to be a second princess. Isaac was again sworn to secrecy.

On this occasion the Duke of Northumberland requested Isaac to go to Carlisle station. There he would find a lady with an injured ankle who was in need of his services. He was requested not to ask the lady her name, but he would be well rewarded for his services. She was a very gracious lady, with several ladies in waiting in a superb carriage.

After examining her ankle, Isaac soon had the damage repaired.

After this incident, it was generally assumed that she was another daughter of the Queen, who had sustained an injury to her ankle, and had limped for some time, the ladies of the court doing likewise, developing what became known as the fashionable limp.

After Isaac's visit to Carlisle station to attend this lady, the fashionable limp disappeared.

Another version of the same event is written as follows:

> On one occasion Isaac received a call to attend a lady at a well-known railway junction. He found his patient in a first-class carriage, shunted on to a siding, surrounded by attendants, male and female, all dressed in plain attire, for the identity of the sufferer was not to be divulged. He examined his patient. Hip trouble, of some duration, and sadly mismanaged. He did what he could, but gave little hope of a permanent cure. He was

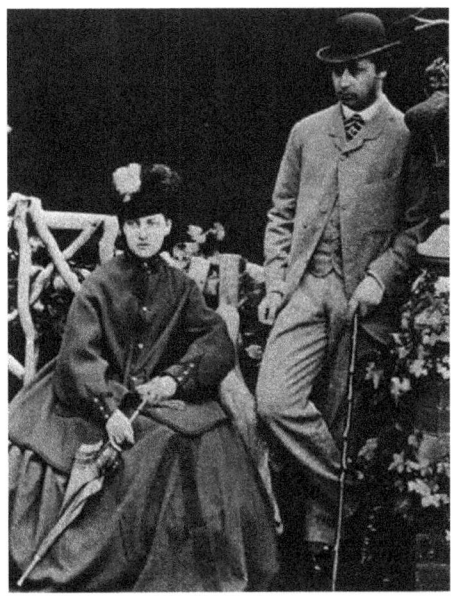 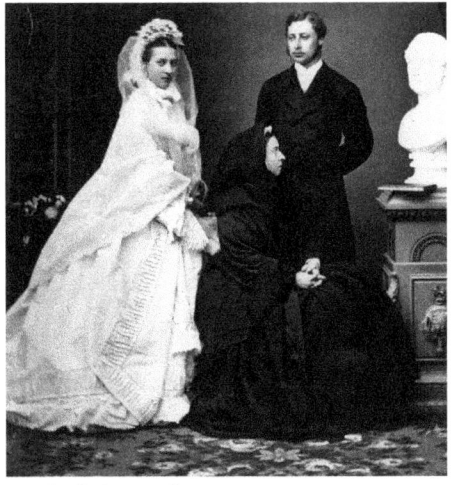

20, left / 21, above. Princess Alexandra with the Prince of Wales 1863.

liberally rewarded. It was currently believed that the patient was none other than the then Princess of Wales who was at the time suffering from a like complaint and walked with a limp to the day of her death.

Princess Alexandra of Denmark became Princess of Wales on the 10th March 1863 and was married to Queen Victoria's son and heir apparent Albert Edward. During the birth of her third child in 1867, Alexandra developed rheumatic fever which threatened her life, and left her with a permanent limp. According to Georgina Battiscombe, a British biographer, specializing mainly in lives from the Victorian era, writes in her book called Queen Alexandra (PR11) that the princess was only able to walk with the help of two walking sticks for a while after this illness.

This would have been tough for an active woman who had previously enjoyed horse riding, hunting, dancing and ice skating.

Edward Keith the Wallington Hall head gardener described Isaac in his book Memories of Wallington Hall as a:

"*rough customer and hard drinker who spent many years of usefulness to the community*".

In his cups at Morpeth and when twitted about his non-cure of Royalty he used to say:

> "A princess without her robes was the same as a pit-wife without her duds. Nature fashioned all folks alike."

Keith's book is based on a recollection of conversations with Sir George Otto Trevelyn who was the Wallington Hall owner from 1886 – 1928.

Despite extensive research and correspondence with Windsor Castle where Queen Victoria's records are held, and enquiries with Alnwick Castle archives I have not been able to find any documents to substantiate the above royal tales - the exact dates of these events is therefore unknown. A good guess would be when Isaac was in his late 60s early 70s based on his photograph possibly holding a Royal command and the known date of his marriage to his second wife Elizabeth. My main intention of this collection of stories is to raise awareness and maybe some learned historian might uncover some hard facts and possibly a letter from Buckingham Palace !

Enquiries with the Royal Archives at Windsor in 2005 produced the following response:

> "I have made a search of our relevant indexes, but I regret that I cannot find any reference to your ancestor Isaac Milburn.
>
> Furthermore I cannot find any indication in our records that Princess Beatrice suffered any injury to her hip from the time of her birth in 1857 until 1886, when Isaac Milburn died."

I personally love the story and think Isaac kept the visits and names relatively secret to a trusted few which would gain him respect and possibly repeat business amongst his royal patients. There is nothing written in the press or adverts during his life about any royal encounters and even the well written detailed obituaries do not mention any specific royal connections. I believe the "knowledge" of the royal events became more widespread after his death but I'm probably biased and would love to be proved wrong.

So no hard and fast evidence from the archives and lots of questions still remain – was there a cover up by the royal medical establishment to hide their limitations of the time?

Some might also believe that the story was complete fiction and a clever marketing ruse by Isaac?

Did Isaac keep the visits secret within a close circle of family members and friends?

The jury is still out despite there being a lot of written and spoken recollections of the events.

We have conflicting tales of a royal visit, two hip injuries one cure and one non cure – the precise detail lost (for the moment) in the passing of time. Tales of being sworn to secrecy and I guess the possibility of treason being in the minds of some might be taking this a little too far in today's line of thinking but maybe this was not the case in Victorian times. I find a plot by the royal surgeons to find out about Isaac's skills and then concealing his success by means of secrecy very intriguing and thought provoking.

And, finally, to the tale involving gunpowder uncovered by Mary Kipling's research and retold as follows:

'Isaac was not without his sense of humour … and at the time was friendly with the village blacksmith in Longhoughton, who one day was relating to Isaac the mysterious disappearance of some of his cartwheels. However much he tried, he had been unable to locate the culprit.

"Well" said Isaac *"there's one way to find out"*

Taking a knife, he hollowed out one of the spokes and placed inside a little dynamite, which he sealed over. They found the culprit alright when a woman had her fireplace blown out !!'

I stand to be corrected but I suspect gunpowder was used instead of dynamite which was not invented until 1880 and would normally need a detonator to produce an explosion. Gunpowder would certainly have been readily available from gun supplier stockists which Isaac would have been familiar with from his gamekeeping days. Explosives would also be available nearby as they were used in the local Longhoughton whinstone and limestone quarries producing kerb stones and lime by means of lime kilns for farming.

The Census records from 1861 to 1881 show that the Robinson family were the Longhoughton village master blacksmiths during this time. William and his son George are noted in the 1861 document and by 1881 George, his two sons and his nephew are all employed in the trade.

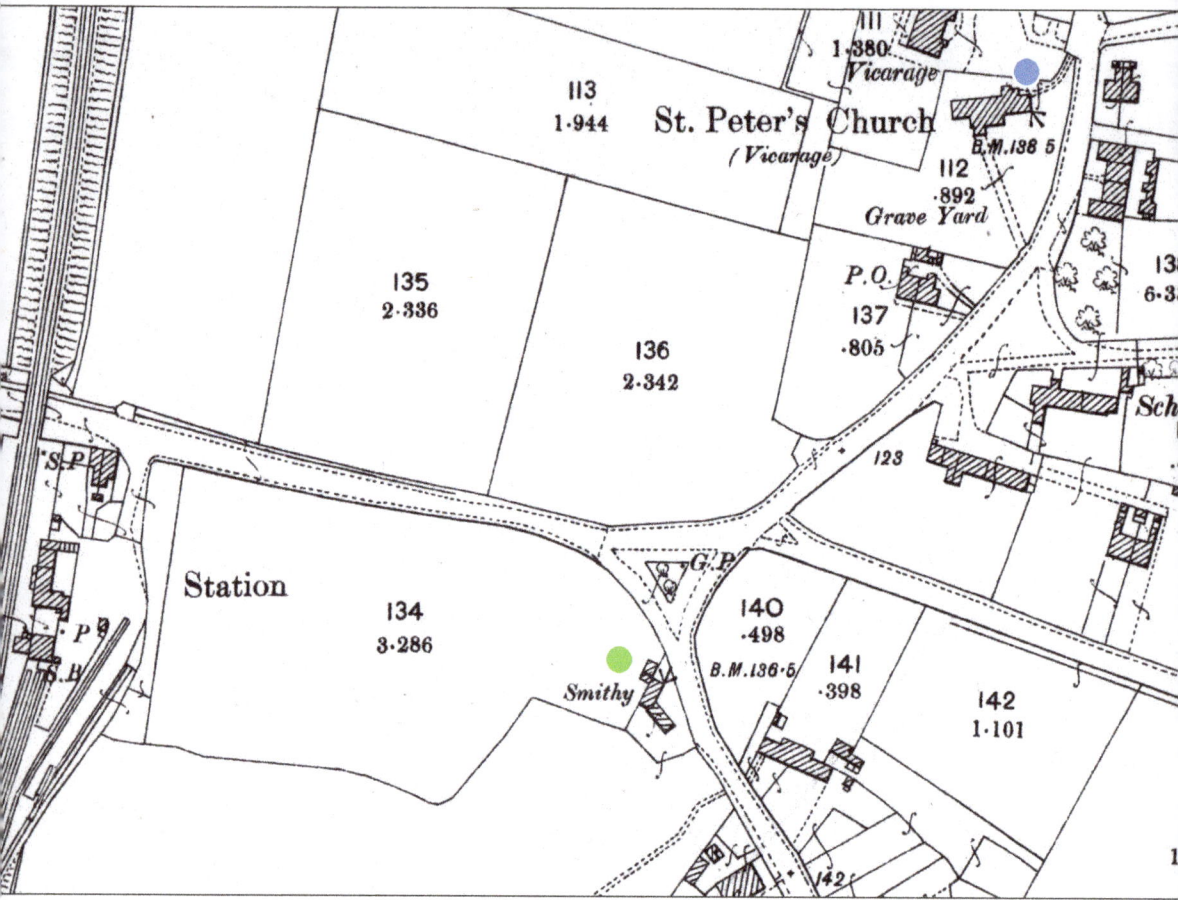

22. Longhoughton Smithy, station and church, 1897.

🟢 Blacksmith 🔵 Isaac Milburn's grave

CHAPTER 6
TESTIMONIAL

It would appear that even in his early 70s Isaac was teaching others keen to learn the art of bonesetting, as an advert appears in the Newcastle Guardian and Tyne Mercury on Saturday 19th October 1867.

Thomas Anderson, Low Spen, Winlanton, Bonesetter will attend Mr J. Routledges Commercial Inn Consett commencing on Saturday Oct 19 and on every alternate Saturday from 10 o'clock till 2pm. Taught under Mr Isaac Milburn Bonesetter upwards of 52 years standing Alnwick Northumberland.

Winlanton and Consett are both south east of Newcastle and out of Isaac's main Alnwick and Morpeth catchment area within central Northumberland. Presumably this was an arrangement that prevented any nearby competition for Isaac.

Isaac's own living conditions at the time were not ideal, as the following article describes and this may have partly led to his testimonial.

An article in the Alnwick Mercury Saturday 6th September 1873 by the Alnwick Rural Sanitary Authority gives us some details of a survey of the Longhoughton district which includes Longbank and describes "Drive Cottage" Isaacs house at the time.

Site of Old Tilesheds

Isaac Milburn the venerable Bonesetter (now age 79) and his wife reside in a brick two storied cottage at the junction of the Longhoughton and Lesbury road with the old Boulmer Road which is now closed and reserved as a "private drive". The porous bricks of the house admit rain and his walls are damp. He obtains drinking water from a cavity under a duck pond. He was invalided at the date of my visit but I have since seen him pursuing his usual professional vocations.

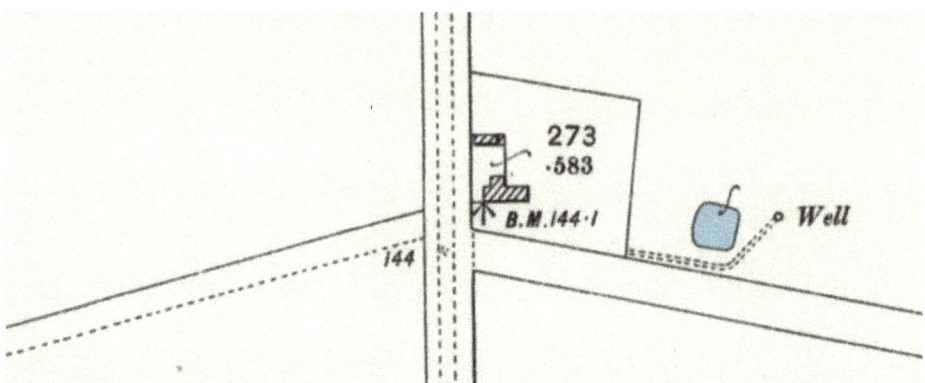

23. Drive Cottage, Tilesheds - Isaac's last home south of Longbank, Longhoughton. Longhouton Ordnance Survey Map 25 inch, 1892–1914.

Six years later in 1879 it was thought that Isaac's services to the public were deserving of some further recognition, and accordingly, a number of gentlemen in and around Alnwick, started a subscription that was responded to from all quarters.

An advert on the 25th January in the Morpeth Herald read as follows:

TESTIMONIAL TO MR ISAAC MILBURN Bonesetter

At a meeting held in Alnwick on Jan 16th 1879 it was unanimously resolved that a Testimonial be presented to Isaac Milburn Bonesetter in appreciation of the valuable services rendered by him.

Mr Milburn is now 84 years of age and it is felt that the benefit derived by the community (for upwards of 50 years) from his skill and experience deserves some recognition at the hands of the public.

Subscriptions will be received by the Treasurer Mr R.T.Grey Lambtons Bank Alnwick by the secretaries and by the committee.

Joseph Archbold Secretary
A.S.Cockburn Secretary
Members of the Committee
Mr Adam Robertson Alnwick
Mr John Bell Alnwick
Mr Jos J Cockburn Alnwick
F.Clark Alnwick
Jas Riddell Alnwick
Ed Allen Alnwick
P Thomson Alnwick
W. Bell Alnwick
Dr Main Alnwick
Mr Jno Jas Horsley Alnwick
Thos Grey Harlow Hill
A Davidson Golden Moor
Robt Donkin Rothbury
The Mayor of Morpeth
R. Wilkinson (Woods & Co) Morpeth
John Brown Bedlington
Thos Embleton auctioneer Berwick.

No doubt the committee members were admirers of Isaac's work and possibly also patients.

A detailed newspaper biography also appeared on March 28th 1879 in the Newcastle Courant as part of the movement to raise awareness of his testimonial and encourage donations from Northumberland, Newcastle and further afield.

After a considerable amount of coaxing, Isaac now aged 84, was encouraged to sit for his photograph at the Alnwick establishment of Mr John Marshall.

An advert dated the 16th June 1880 describes the photographer's business as follows:

Artist and Photographer 22, Bondgate without Alnwick - all the latest improvements in photography - "an enlarged photograph finished in oils" - offering Alnwick a portrait club by subscription. Established 1860. Portraits taken daily, dull weather no object.

The invitation to the testimonial reads as follows:

"Isaac Milburn Testimonial

The presentation, consisting of a portrait, and a Purse of Gold, will be made on Thursday the 31st July at six O'clock in the evening, in the Nags Head Inn, Alnwick, when all subscribers and friends will be invited to attend. A dinner will be provided on the occasion, Tickets 2s.6d. each may be got from Mr F.Clark, Nags Head Inn, or from secretaries, not later than the 29th July."

Tickets costing 2 shillings and sixpence each in 1879 would be the equivalent of approximately £15 in 2020 UK currency.

The Berwickshire News and General Advertiser mentions on Tuesday the 5th August 1879 that "A public dinner was held in Alnwick on Thursday night at which Mr Isaac Milburn the well known bonesetter was presented with his portrait and a purse of money. Mr Milburn suitably acknowledged the gift."

The front book cover portrait of Isaac is unsigned so this is possibly the photograph mentioned above finished in oils by John Marshall.

Isaac travelled to Lesbury in 1880 on the occasion of the general election in order to record his vote for Earl Percy.

A few years later on Saturday 11th Feb 1882 the York Herald mentions another area of Isaac's work.

Mr M Morrison whose Waterloo Cup nomination has been returned to the committee intends retiring from coursing. His old dog Free Flag who injured himself at Gosforth has had his stifle joint reset by Isaac Milburn the bonesetter.

Waterloo coursing meeting Wednesday 15th Feb 1882
64 subscriptions @ £25 each. Total purse £1600
£500 winner 2nd £200

The complex stifle joint in the hind limbs of a horse and dog is the equivalent of the human knee and joins three bones: the femur, patella, and tibia.

There is a newspaper advert dated 7th June 1884 showing a change of pub for Isaac's surgeries from the Black Bull to the premises next door called the New Phoenix Inn in Morpeth for Wednesday consultations.

His work was continuous week after week, year after year and there are newspaper adverts stating that he will be working and travelling to Alnwick and Morpeth right up to the 30th August 1884, when he was 90 !!

On 6th September 1884 an advert appears mentioning that Isaac "will not be present at Alnwick or Morpeth but may be consulted at any time at his residence in Longbank within 10 minutes walk of Longhoughton station"

On Saturday Nov 5th 1885 The Alnwick and County Gazette printed an article as follows:

> "We have missed from amongst us a very familiar character and many will learn with revived interest that Isaac Milburn the bonesetter of almost national notoriety is still living at Longbank near Longhoughton. Though his health is naturally failing he continues at the patriarchal age of 91 to practice his humane art with a skill and precision truly marvellous.
>
> His bent figure and crabbed face are too well known to require description and all acquainted with him know that under a somewhat gruff exterior lies a kindly and sympathetic heart, while all who have placed their suffering limbs in his hands have found that in them hands are combined the soft and gentle touch of a woman with an almost magic dexterity of manipulation. Isaac has been married twice and his second wife a hale dame of 70 is his sole companion in his red brick house at Longbank. He continues to operate on a constant stream of patients who have much faith in his magic powers."

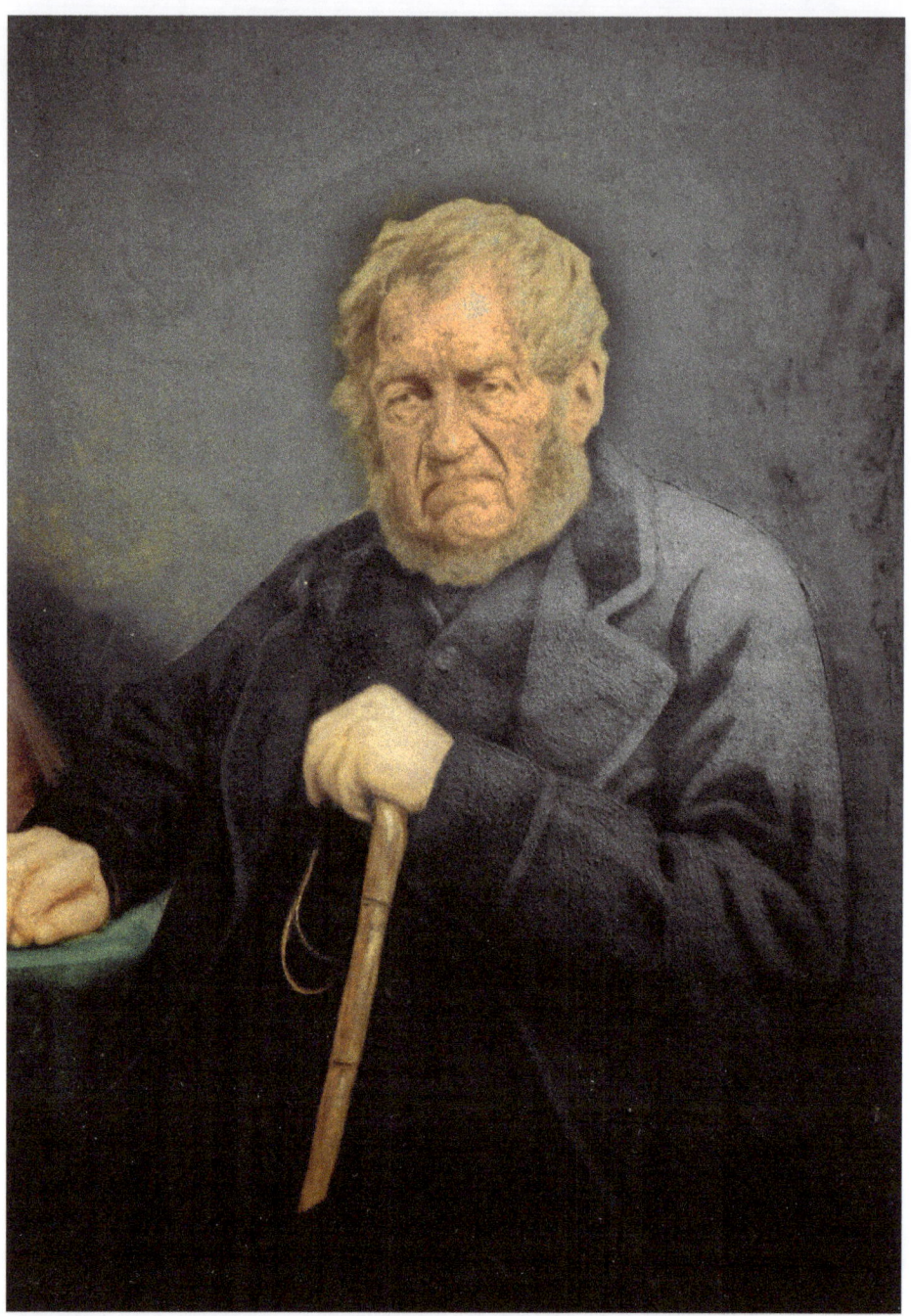

24. Oil Portrait of Isaac.

CHAPTER 7
DEATH OF ISAAC MILBURN

Isaac died on the 30th January 1886 aged 92 years old, at Drive Cottage, Longbank, Longhoughton. His death certificate gives the cause of death as "softening of brain 2 years", certified by Alex. Jas. Main M.D. and his wife Margaret was present at his death.

A lengthy obituary was written in the Newcastle Courant and a public subscription was raised for a memorial fund by a public notice in the Morpeth Herald on Saturday 3rd April 1886 as follows:

ISAAC MILBURN MEMORIAL FUND

At a public meeting, held at the Nags Head Inn Alnwick on March 31st a subscription list was opened for the purpose of erecting a memorial stone in memory of the late Isaac Milburn.

Subscriptions will be gladly received by the following:

Editor Morpeth Herald
Editor Alnwick Guardian
Editor Alnwick & County Gazette
Editor Newcastle Courant
Mr James Grey Low Stead Lesbury
Mr F Clark Alnmouth
Mr Dodds Longhoughton
Mr Jos Archbold Honorary Secretary
Mr A.S. Cockburn Honorary Secretary

The winning bid for the headstone work was from Danial McMillan described in the Alnwick Mercury newspaper as a stone cutter, monumental sculptor located in Dispensary Street Alnwick.

Alnwick monumental works, headstones, tombs, marble tablets, fountains, vases, lettering done neatly in town and country.

A notice in the Morpeth Herald on Saturday 28th May 1887 advises that a memorial stone to Isaac Milburn the bonesetter to be viewed at the studio of Mr Danial McMillan.

On the same day The Shields Daily News (PR12) prints the following article:

> "Memorial to the late Isaac Milburn – a very fine example of monumental art, unique in design, to perpetuate the memory of the late Isaac Milburn of Longbank, renowned as a bonesetter, throughout the north of England, and whose name is familiar in almost every household, has just been produced from the chisel of Mr Danial McMillan of Alnwick, whose skill and genius as a sculptor have contributed so much towards the adornment of most churchyards and cemeteries in the northern counties with chaste memorials of regard and affection for departed friends and relatives.

The memorial being the spontaneous tribute of the friends and admirers of "Old Isaac" the work was offered for competition and Mr McMillan was entrusted with it by the committee, the monument is unexampled in the neighbourhood. It is a large monolith of purest marble from the famous quarries of Carrara.

It is 2 foot six inches x 3 foot six inches and weighs about 2 tons and has been dressed with great skill to represent a pyramid of rugged storm beaten rocks (13 in number) typical of old Isaac's life. On the front of the pile nicely cut from the solid, and secured as it were by a tastefully – wrought tendril of ivy with leaves to the face of the stone, is a scroll bearing the following dedicatory inscription in imperishable characters.

> "Erected in token of gratitude in memory of Isaac Milburn bonesetter, who died at Longbank Jan 30th 1886 aged 92."

The memorial is at present to be seen in McMillan's yard in Dispensary Street, but will shortly be placed on the grave of "Old Isaac" in the rural churchyard at Longhoughton.

A very excellent photograph of the stone has been taken by Mr John Hikely Alnwick.

In 1967 Isaac's life was depicted in a painting by Mary Kipling. Mary as mentioned previously spent a considerable amount of time researching Isaac's life and was able to obtain his likeness from an old faded photograph loaned to her by a lady living near Morpeth, whose grandmother was Isaac's daughter Jane. The small scenes in the painting show different episodes in his life, from working with his father as a joiner and cartwright, Wallington Hall, Bolt Cottage and then onto Drive Cottage. Mary was able to visit all the places portrayed in the painting to do her drawings and upon her request to the National Trust permission was given to use her drawings of Wallington. The rabbits at the bottom of the picture, represent his work as a gamekeeper and also the knowledge he received from them.

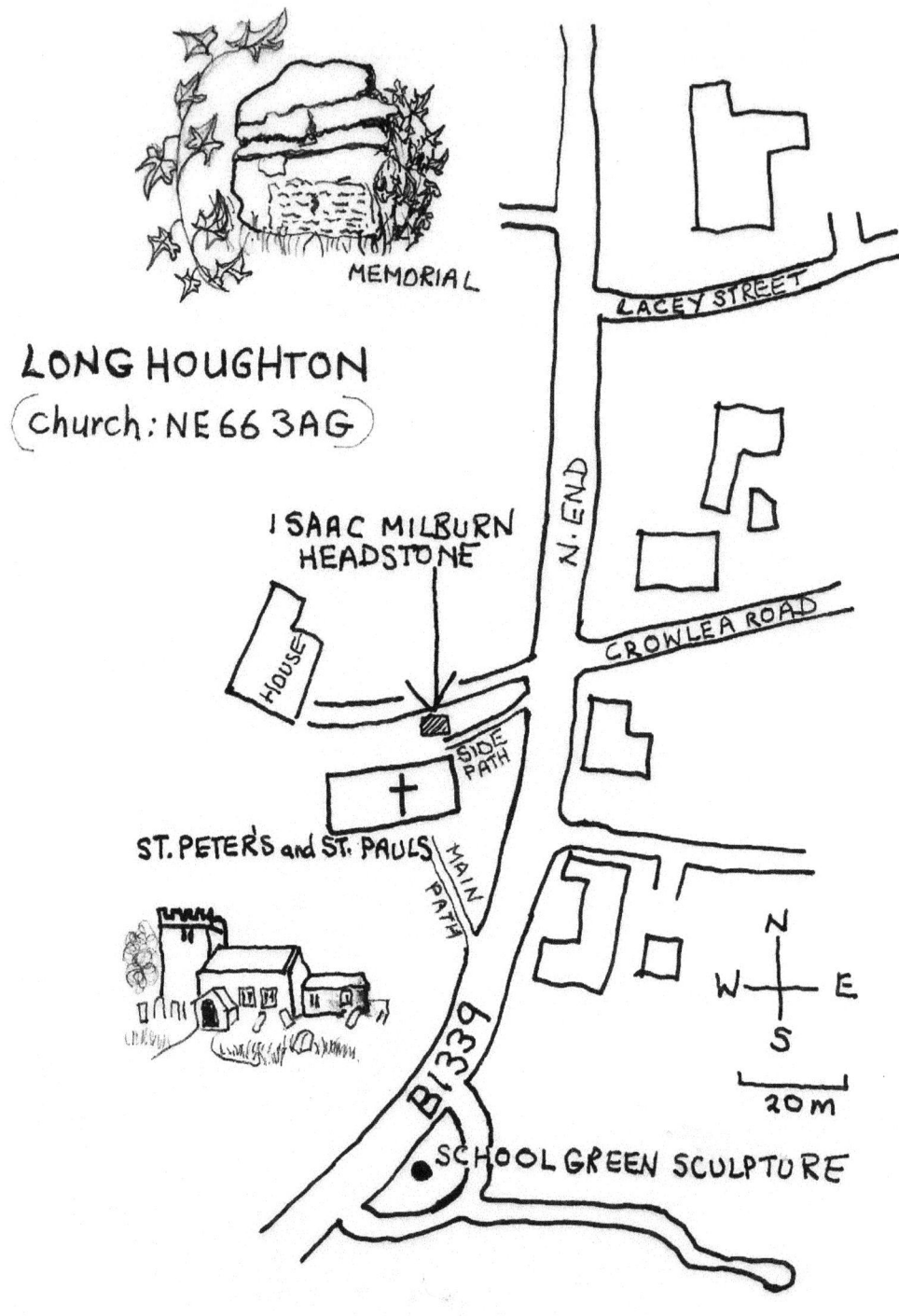

25. St. Peter and St. Paul church map.

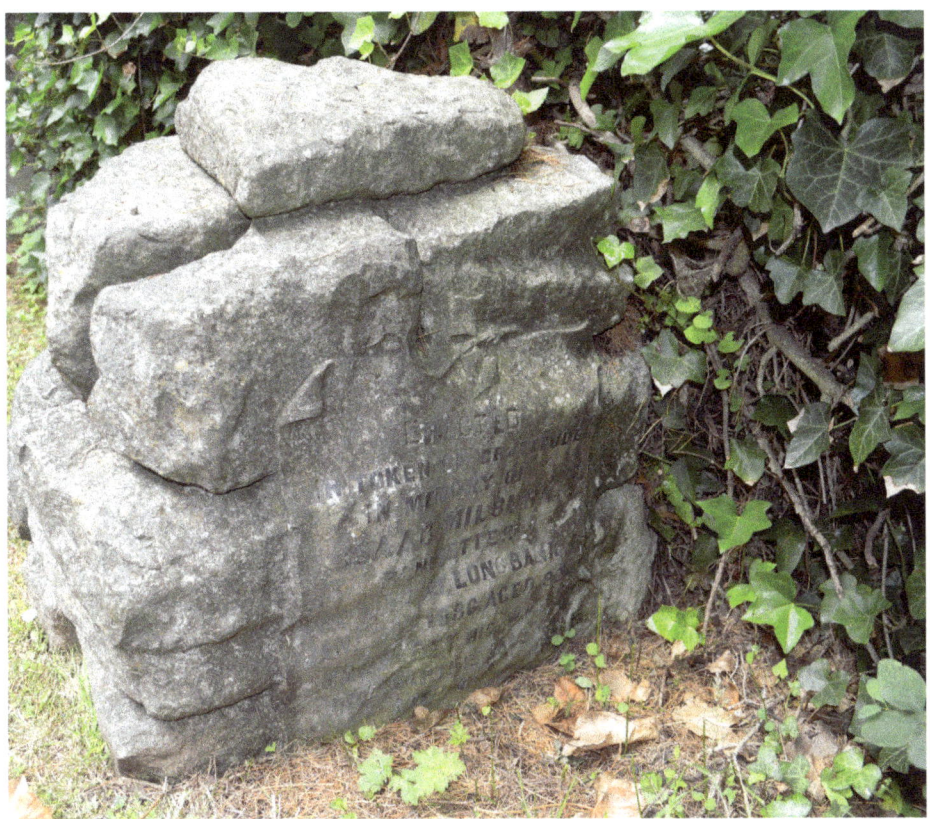
26. Isaac memorial headstone at the east end of Longhougton church.

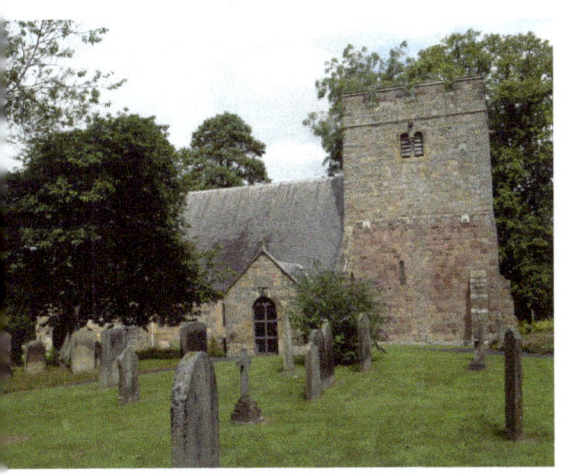
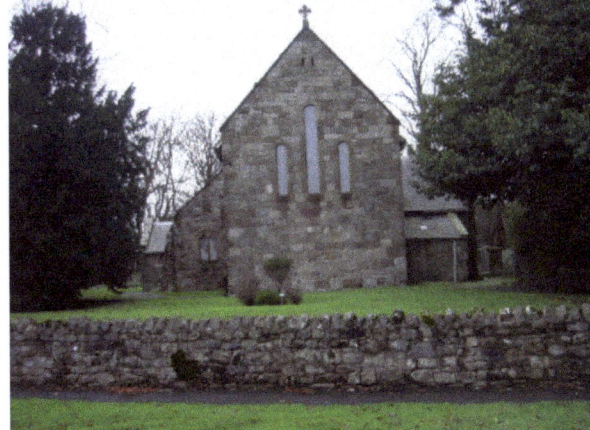
27a / 27b. St. Peter and St. Paul church - south / east view.

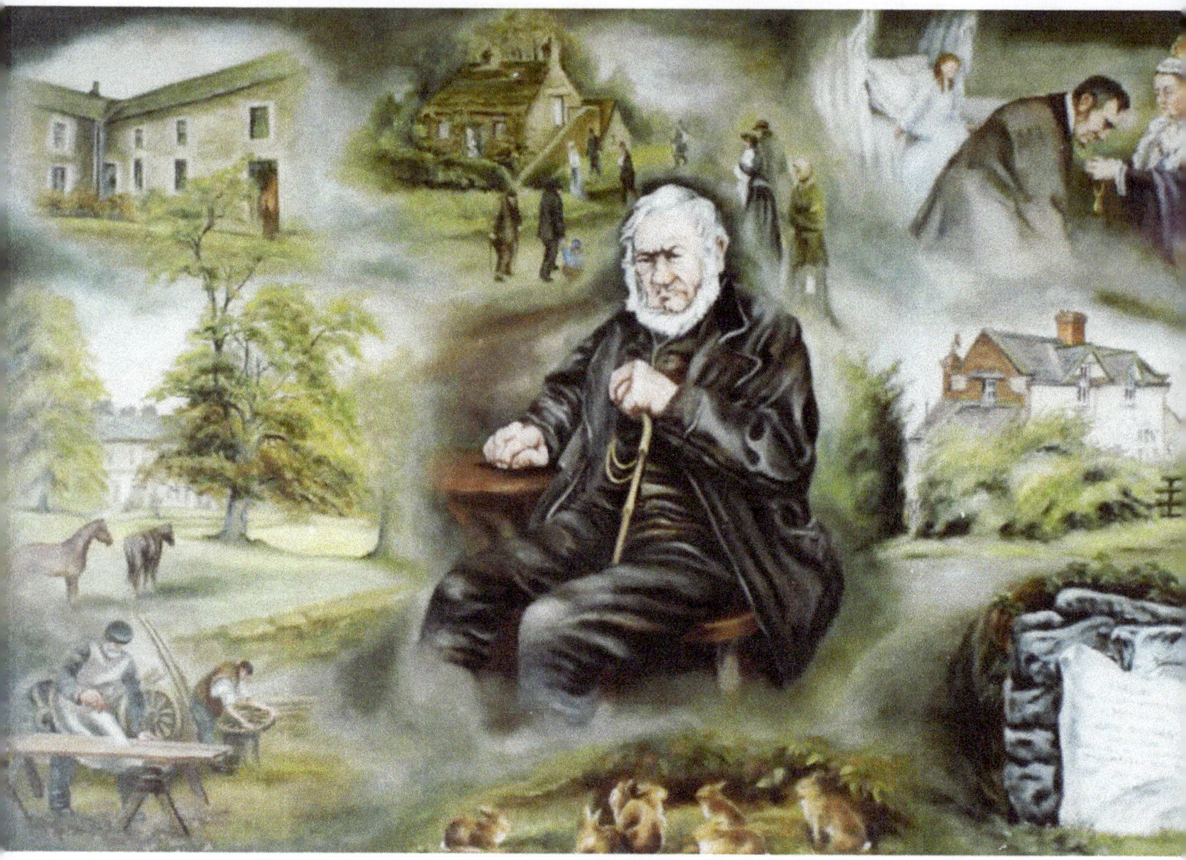

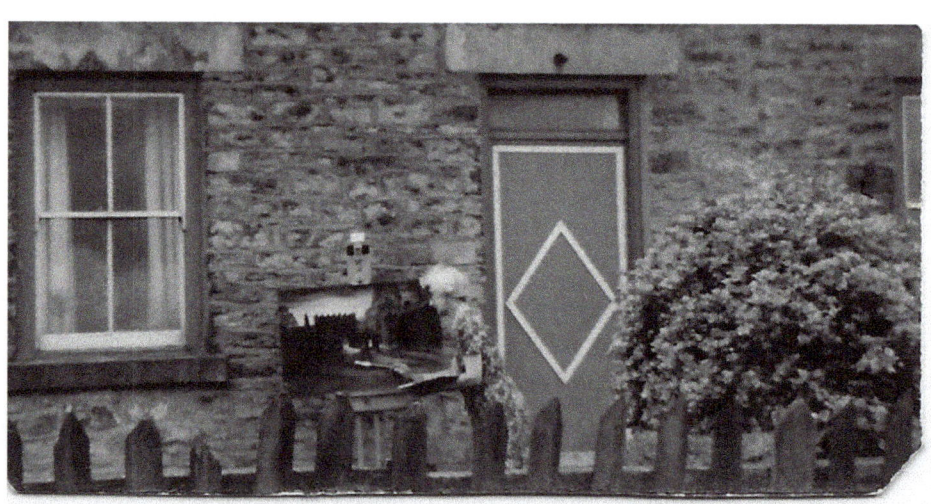

28 / 29. Painting by Mary Kipling and the artist herself painting outside her house at Consett.

CHAPTER 8
CONTROVERSY

Not unsurprisingly after such an eventful life, Isaac's story does not end at his death, his obituary in the Newcastle Courant kicking off a bit of a storm.

The Newcastle Courant was established in 1711 and continued weekly for 135 years. In February 1876, The Newcastle Courant merged with The Newcastle Journal, which had changed from a weekly to a daily newspaper in December 1860.

Christopher S. Jeaffreson F.R.C.S (Fellow of the Royal College of Surgeons), Saville Row, Newcastle-on-Tyne writes a letter to the Newcastle Courant in response to Isaac's obituary. The term 'surgeon' is traditionally described as a person who performed operations with the use of surgical instruments. Some surgeons however, particularly in the 19th century, also worked in other areas of medical practice. Note I have taken the liberty of explaining in the glossary some of the words in his letter as I had no idea of their meaning and my impression is that this "learned" gentlemen obviously wanted the reader to know he had a distinct level of education. His first letter is as follows:

> *Sir, - Kindly allow me space to make a few comments upon the two columns of panegyric on the life and works of the deceased bonesetter, named Isaac Milburn, published in your issue of Monday last. Upon the principle of de mortuus nil nisi bonum, I should have preferred remaining silent; but an article such as you have published is so misleading, calculated to do so much injury to the ignorant portion of the public and withal such an outrage upon a science which, within late years, has shown such strong*

claims to be classified amongst the exact sciences, that it cannot be allowed to pass without challenge or remark.

To maintain that an uneducated man who has been brought up as a gamekeeper, and past the best years of his life as a village publican, who has never dissected a human limb in his life, who is ignorant of anatomy, and who acquired his first knowledge of fracture, dislocations, and other injuries by practising upon hares, rabbits, and other four footed beasts, whose construction differs widely from the human frame; whilst provoking only a smile of derisive contempt in educated and thoughtful persons, tends to the perpetuation amongst ignorant persons of many ideas, prejudices and superstitious beliefs, which it should be the object of an enlightened press to correct and dispel.

Your sketch presents the history of Isaac Milburn's life and work as written by a friend and admirer. The mystery which surrounds most of the tales there related, provokes one's suspicion to their genuineness, and in many instances stronger language might be used to describe some of them.

I am far from saying that, in some instances, he may not have done some good – shots fired at random will sometimes hit the mark – but if the history of Mr Milburn were written by the profession of this district, quite a different light would be thrown upon the practice of bone-setting, as carried out by ignorant and uneducated persons; and it would present a sorry chapter of the blind credulity of a large section of the public. I could myself, personally, furnish instances in which his incalculable injuries were inflicted by his ignorant manipulations, and I have little doubt these instances might be multiplied into hundreds and thousands if other medical men were to relate their experiences, - I am, &c., C.S.JEAFFRESON F.R.C.S.

There would seem to be a huge rift between some of the qualified health profession and the traditional bonesetters. Both parties with different skill sets of knowledge and experience, both with the same aim in mind trying to alleviate suffering of the common man. Remember this is before any National Health Service, which started in 1952 and prior to this doctors and bonesetters would have charged patients accordingly. I guess doctors and surgeons would be trying to establish their credentials after years of study and bonesetters might in some cases be considered as lower cost competition. Bonesetters would however be more accessible to the hard-pressed working man and woman with limited income.

Anyway the battle of words continued with a retort from the obituary writer:

> *Sir,- I am glad that the sketch of Isaac Milburn has attracted the attention of the medical profession. By Mr Jeaffreson you are charged with having, in admitting the sketch in your columns, done what an enlightened press ought not to do; I am charged, as a friend and admirer of Isaac, with having written a panegyric on the deceased bonesetter. You need none of my help in rebutting the charge made against your editorial capacity and enlightenment. As for myself, I could not lay claim to Isaac's friendship, having seen him not more than half-a-dozen times, and spoken to him only once. Personal interest in him or his neither has, nor had, any existence or influence in the production of the sketch. So much for friendship and panegyric. As for Mr Jeaffreson's "suspicion of the genuineness" of the tales, all, except two, are recorded from my own personal knowledge. The two out of my individual ken are the visit to London (Princess Beatrice) and to the (Royal) saloon railway carriage (Princess Alexandra) ; these are so current throughout Northumberland, and so firmly believed in, that no sketch of the old man's career would have been complete without them. Mr Jeaffreson has not read carefully. Instead of saying that Isaac got his first knowledge of fractures and dislocations by practising on hares, rabbits, &c., I was careful to describe those tales as apocryphal. Having thus vindicated the sketch from the charges made against it by your correspondent, it is only necessary to add that any man whose work increases in popularity over a period of seventy years, as did Isaac's, cannot be written down as an ignorant quack. Quacks with or without qualifications, do not sustain their reputation for anything like so lengthened a time. Mr Charles Waterton, the Yorkshire traveller and naturalist, who was neither an ignorant nor uneducated person, entertained very different opinions respecting men like Isaac Milburn from those of Mr Jeaffreson, and, as he no doubt knows, Mr Waterton was an authority on the subject. – I am, &c.,*
> THE WRITER OF THE ARTICLE.

Another letter to the Courant and the Alnwick and County Gazette on February 6th to support Isaac and the obituary writer is by Fergus Clark who by all accounts was an assistant and a very close friend of Isaac's.

The Late Isaac Milburn

Sir, Having read in Wednesday morning Journal, a letter signed C.S.JEFFERSON F.R.C.S. commenting upon the deceased bonesetter Isaac Milburn and attempting to throw doubt upon the authenticity of the cases he is reported to have successfully dealt with. I beg to state that they are substantially correct and if necessary I can relate hundreds more of such cases to which I can bear testimony as an eyewitness. I have known Isaac Milburn personally for the last forty years and attended with him in all parts of the country for the last twelve years of his practice and I can produce the names of hundreds of patients who can testify to the benefit they received at the hands of the deceased bonesetter. If the learned F.R.C.S. can produce the name of one who has, as he says, suffered from Isaac's want of skill I will find fifty for every such one, who has been successfully operated upon. He confesses that Isaac "may have done some good" as "shots fired at random will sometimes hit the mark" but what about the many learned surgeons who have fired random shots in this direction and missed the mark? Yours & c, Fergus Clark Alnmouth Feb 3rd, 1886.

Mr Jeaffreson was not going to sit back at this repost and wrote the following:

TO THE EDITOR OF THE "Newcastle Daily Journal"

Sir, - I observe that in your issue of Thursday, a gentleman from Alnwick writes, and gives what he is pleased to term "a flat denial" to most of the facts contained in my letter of February the 3rd. From the confidence with which he speaks of Mr Milburn's success, and the ocular testimony he has had of his skill, I was led, at first to think my critic was some medical man in disguise; or some secede who had abandoned the legitimate ranks of the profession to follow the teachings and practice of the self taught son of Aesculapius, and that his opinion might have some weight in the matters medical and surgical. I therefore instituted a careful search in the Medical Directory for the name of "Fergus Clark." Not being successful in this direction, I then turned to the Post Office Directory, and found that gentleman of that name was the proprietor of an ancient hostelry known by the name of the "Nags Head." Now if I am right in presuming that this gentleman is the

self-appointed arbiter upon matters purely medical and surgical, few will think me wrong in declining to enter upon any discussion with him, and many will think me right in the advice which I am now about to give, viz.: that the sign of the "Nags Head" should be taken down, and in its place should be substituted that of a humbler, though closely allied four-footed animal.- I am, &c.
C.S.JEAFFERSON.

The 1881 Census records Mr Jeafferson as living at 2, Fernwood Road, Jesmond with his wife Constance, three children, a page and three servants.

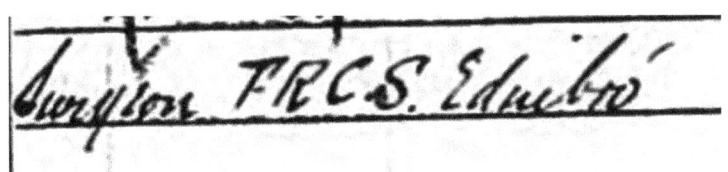

30. Census record.

His occupation is listed as a "surgeon" and "FRCS" (Fellow of the Royal College of Surgeons) and what looks like "Edinbro" so probably Edinburgh.

More letters of support for Isaac appear in the press on the 4th Feb:

Sir, - With reference to the respective claims of the medical profession, and bonesetters, as qualified to successfully perform, in many cases, the dangerous (as to malformation) process of bone-setting, will you allow me give two cases, which I can personally vouch for, as they happened in my own family?

<u>Dancing Child</u>

My wife, when a child, had her arm dislocated by a relative falling upon her while dancing, and after being treated for over two months by a local medical man of undoubted ability as a doctor, with not the slightest benefit (in fact the child was in continual agony of pain, and could not move her arm in the slightest), a change of air was recommended, and she was sent to the neighbourhood of Alnwick, and while there, her father was induced to take her to "old Isaac Milburn" who, as luck happened, they met on the road, and not being aware of the identity of their informant, gruffly said that he was...

"the beast",

on inquiry to his abode.

To cut my story short, the child was taken to a neighbouring cottage, and within three days was able to lift her arm, and in a week to use it.

Toddler's Fall

The second case was that of my little girl, 18 months old, who had her shoulder dislocated, and the collar bone nearly, but not quite broken, through a fall from a careless girl's shoulder in July last year. The child was attended for a broken collar bone by a local medical gentleman (who knew nothing about the dislocated shoulder) for three weeks, and at the end of that time, the poor little thing not being able to move her arm in the slightest degree – and in continual pain – I was induced to get the services of Mr Storey, a bonesetter of Deckham Gateshead, and the next day – in fact, to be precise, 10 minutes after the operation, which did not occupy more than three or four seconds – the child's arm was in normal condition, and she was able to use it perfectly. I need say no more, excepting that in my own case and in several more I can mention, I am thoroughly convinced that the majority of doctors may understand the theoretical, but certainly not the practical side of bone-setting. – I am, &c., "J. H." Gateshead, Feb 4th, 1886.

Another supportive response by letter to the press was as follows:

Sir, - Dr C.S. Jeaffreson, F.R.S.'s comments on the late Isaac Milburn in your issue of the 3rd inst. are calculated to do a great deal of injury to those who have acquired the art of bone-setting. He says Isaac has not studied the anatomy of the body. Probably not. Doctors have; and yet they will set a leg when it is dislocated for a broken leg. I have suffered from such.

Kicking Horse

I get my leg dislocated by the kick of a horse in Newcastle, and was taken to the head doctors who instantly said: "oh, your leg is broken." I submitted to his opinion; and he put on two large splints and tied them tightly with about 100 yards of bandages, the result being that the pain increased until I could not suffer it any longer. With the assistance of a friend I got them off and fomented well with hot water, and sent for a lady bonesetter (Mrs Weight, 19, Gibson Street), who instead of treating it for a broken leg, put the knee-cap on and gave me liniment to allay the pain and reduce the swelling. So much for bonesetters. I can also testify to the abilities of Isaac. I have unfortunately had my bones dislocated seven times – legs, arms, fingers, &c. – and have also been put right by Isaac. Thousands of others can say the same respecting Isaac's abilities as a successful bonesetter.

<u>Herring Smoker</u>

I saw an instance of a doctor's skill in bone-setting a few months ago. A young man who, whilst working at his trade as a herring smoker, fell and hurt his arm in Scotland. He went to a doctor, who set it for a broken arm. And put it together nicely with splints, sending him home to North Sunderland. As soon as I saw it I said, "Your arm is only out." He took my advice and went to Isaac, who gave the doctor his usual "blessings," and put the joint in, and in a few weeks the young man was able to go back to his work. Doctors are useful for the salts and senna business, but do not understand bone-setting. – I am, &c., "W. G." North Sunderland.

A final letter of support was printed and written by an Edward Liddle from Gateshead.

Sir, - To many hundreds of people who knew the late Isaac Milburn and his work a feeling of indignation must have arisen within them when they read the scurrilous letter of Dr Jeaffreson of Newcastle, as published in the Journal. Evidently the doctor rushed into print respecting a man about whom he absolutely knew nothing, or else he had an unbounded prejudice against him. Here was a man above 90 years of age, who commenced the practice and study of bone-setting when quite a young man, and who until very recently had a very much larger practice than the whole of Newcastle combined – his patients numbered many scores each month (from all parts of England) – and yet we are to believe, according to Dr Jeaffreson, that this man was entirely ignorant of anatomy ! A gross libel !

If ever a man was master of the subject it was Isaac, although he could not boast of the technical names belonging to it. He was familiar with every ligament, tendon, or sinew in the body as with every bone, even the minutest, in the framework or skeleton to which the fleshy tabernacle is built. If he could have seen the hundreds of people Isaac had through his hands in the course of each year and examined their cases he would not have condemned him, but, on the contrary, would have been inclined to vent his spleen on his brother doctors who had had charge of many of the cases, and who had shown their entire ignorance of the subject. I have known many cases where Isaac effected cures after medical men had failed.

Rod Fisherman

Some fifteen years ago I had the misfortune to injure one of my knees when on a fishing excursion. As soon as I got hobbled to my lodgings I sent for the doctor and after examination he pronounced the injury to be a severe sprain. I came home and the following week I sought the assistance of one of the most eminent men in Newcastle. He ordered the limb to be laid up and gave me a lotion. I was lame – could not bend the knee in walking – and had difficulty when seating myself. There was neither discolouring nor swelling. I got worse, and after about 8 weeks I was advised to visit Milburn. I went, and in an instant I was told that " a leader was wrong." In five minutes I was walking across the room without any assistance. This surely was a lucky shot "fired at random."

I also had him at my house for a dislocated shoulder. In a few minutes the patient was enabled to move her arm where she wished, and there was no further trouble with the shoulder.

Goose Lady

A few days before Christmas,1884, I went to visit the old man at Long Bank ; and I had not been in his place more than a few minutes when a hamper was brought in, from a lady residing at Reedwater*, containing her annual present of a goose. Inside the hamper was also a note, wishing that Isaac might live many years to continue his good work. This lady about 14 years previously, had injured her hand, and although she had two doctors *they were afraid she would lose it. Isaac put her right – and hence her gratitude. Before Dr Jeaffreson wrote about "ignorant manipulations" – "shots fired at random" – it would have been more becoming if he had kept his name out of print until he had enquired more fully into the history and doing of Isaac Milburn. I am, &c., Edward Liddle. 48, High Street, Gateshead.*

*Reedwater is most likely to be the area around the River Rede, between Otterburn and Redesmouth some 26 miles west of Morpeth where Isaac held his consultations. Reedwater might be a spelling mistake in the press although on old maps there is a Reedswater House and a train station called Reedsmouth Junction. The lady mentioned could quite easily have taken the train from Reedsmouth Junction to Morpeth on the now closed Wansbeck "Wannie" line which passed through Scots Gap and Middleton stations which were near Wallington Hall.

Bone-setting at this time was however attracting the attention of a number of far sighted doctors keen to learn about the superior skill and success of unprofessional men in this department of surgery.

Hunting Gent

A Dr Smailes wrote an account called the "Life of George Moore" in which he writes "the eminent draper and philanthropist sustained an injury to his shoulder by a fall in the hunting field, how the most experienced and learned surgeons in London failed to ascertain the real nature of the hurt and so left him for two years with his arm in a sling, nothing the better but rather the worse, and how at the end of that time Mr Moore was induced to consult an uneducated bonesetter, who at the first examination determined the seat and nature of the mischief and in a brief time had his patient whole and well, enjoying the free and painless use of the long imprisoned limb"

A Dr William Chambers who produced a popular 16 page magazine called Chambers's Edinburgh Journal takes up the question of bone-setting.

He suggests that in interests of suffering humanity, it was desirable to collect so many well – authorized cases of successful bone-setting by amateur or non-professional persons as possible, with the view of removing from people's minds the inherent prejudice against the employment of any but legally qualified surgeons.

Pear Tree Man

Not an Isaac Milburn case but another one in the Courant article that illustrates the skill of the lay bonesetter.

The ability of a local Yorkshire bonesetter has been publicly declared by a man who was peculiarly qualified to appreciate and rightly estimate the skill and sound treatment adopted by him in his own case. This was Charles Waterton, the renowned field naturalist of Walton Hall, Wakefield, an educated gentleman who in many perils had to be on many occasions physician and surgeon to others as well as to himself. His own account of the incident is in this wise. Towards the close of the year 1850" (when he was 78 years of age), "I had reared a ladder, full seven yards long, against a standard pear tree, and I mounted near the top of this ladder, with pruning knife in hand, in order that I might correct an overgrown luxuriance in the tree.

Suddenly the ladder swerved in a lateral direction. I adhered to it manfully, myself and the ladder coming simultaneously to the ground with astounding velocity. There was partial concussion of the brain; and my whole side from head to shoulder felt as though it had been pounded in a mill. Three months after the accident, not withstanding the best surgical skill, my arm showed the appearance of a stiff and withered deformity. And now my general state of health was not as it ought to be; for incessant pain prevented sleep, whilst food itself did little good. But my slumbers were strangely affected. I was eternally fighting with wild beasts. Nine bulldogs attacked me one night in the high road, some of them having the head of a crocodile. I had now serious thoughts about having the arm amputated. This operation was fully resolved upon, when luckily the advice of my trusty gamekeeper, John Ogden, rendered it unnecessary. One morning 'Master,' said he to me, 'I'm sure your going to the grave. You'll die to a certainty. Let me go for the old bonesetter, whose family has exercised the art, from father to son, time out of mind'

On viewing my poor remnant of an arm – 'Your wrist,' said he, 'is sorely injured; a callus having formed betwixt the hand and the arm. The elbow is out of joint, and the shoulder somewhat driven forwards. This last affair will prevent you from raising the arm to your head.' Melancholy look out! 'But you can cure me, doctor ?' said I. 'Yes,' he replied firmly ; 'only let me have my own way ' 'Then take the arm, and with it take the elbow, wrist, and shoulder. I deliver them up to you. Do what you please with them. Pain is no consideration in this case. I dare say I shall have enough of it.' 'You will,' said he emphatically. This resolute bonesetter, who I always compared to Chiron the Centaur for his science and his strength, began his operations like a man of business. In fourteen days, by means of potent embrocations, stretching, pulling, twisting, and jerking, he forced the shoulder and the wrist to obey him, and perform their former healthy movements. The elbow was a complicated affair. It required greater exertions and greater attention. In fact it was a job for Hercules himself. Having done the needful to it, secundum artem for one and twenty days, he seemed satisfied with the progress which he had made and he said quite coolly, 'I'll finish you off this afternoon.' At four o'clock, post- meridian, his bandages, his plasters and his wadding having been placed on the table in regular order, he doffed his coat, tucked his shirt above his elbows, and said that a glass of ale would do him good. 'Then I'll have a glass of soda water with you ' said I; 'and we'll drink each other's health and success to the undertaking'. The remaining act was one of unmitigated severity; but was absolutely necessary. The bonesetter performed his part with resolution scarcely to be contemplated, but which was really required under existing circumstances. Laying hold of the crippled arm just above the elbow with one hand, and below it with the other he smashed to atoms by main force the callus which had formed in the dislocated joint; the elbow itself cracking, as though the interior parts of it had consisted of tobacco pipe shanks. All being now effected as far as force and skill were concerned, the remainder became a mere work of time. So putting a five pound note, by way of extra fee into this sturdy operator's hand, the binding up of this now rectified elbow joint was effected by him, with a nicety and a knowledge truly astonishing. Health soon resumed her ancient right, sleep went hand in hand with a quiet mind, life was once more worth enjoying; and here I am just now, sound as an acorn." Mr Waterton adds that he would have filled volumes with the recital of cases which the same man had brought to a happy conclusion. This bonesetter was Mr John Crowther, who in 1856, had passed his seventy-seventh year, and whose ancestors, for time out of mind, had exercised the art. Testimony like this from such a man as Waterton should be sufficient to ensure the unbelieving that natural aptitude, close observation and study, and long experience put to good profit, are the only secrets in the undoubted skill of Isaac Milburn.

It would seem to be the case that there was ongoing continual discussion, debate and disagreement between doctors about the value of bone-setting throughout the 19th century.

However at this point in history scientists were on the cusp of a remarkable medical breakthrough which would radically and slowly change such controversy in the world of doctors, surgeons and bonesetters.

This was the discovery of X-rays in 1895, nine years on from Isaac's death, by Wilhelm Roentgen, Professor of Physics in Worzburg in Bavaria.

In 1896 an X-ray department was set up at the Glasgow Royal Infirmary, one of the first of its type in the world. Dr John Macintyre head of the department produced a number of x-rays showing kidney stones and a penny in the throat of a child. Later that year Dr Hall-Edwards became one of the first people to use an X-ray to make a diagnosis - he discovered a needle embedded in a woman's hand. During the following twenty years x-rays were used to treat soldiers fighting in the Boer war and those fighting in WWI, finding bone fractures and bullets in soldiers. X-ray machines even started to appear in theatrical side shows until the dangers of regular encounters to X- ray exposure became known.

CHAPTER 9
ISAAC'S LEGACY

We know that a T.W.Atkinson of Morpeth and Fergus Clark of Alnwick were actively assisting Isaac in his later years. T.W. Atkinson continues to work as a bonesetter after Isaac's death and regular adverts start to appear from 1886/7 offering his services on Wednesdays at the house of John Heddon, New Phoenix Hotel in Morpeth hours 11 – 2 as usual and Tuesdays at Miss Browns, Old White Swan Inn, Cloth Market Newcastle 1 to 4pm. The advert mentions he was an assistant for 8 years with Isaac Milburn bonesetter. T.W. Atkinson died on the 1st August 1906 and two of his mourners were his two sons Charles Atkinson and Edward B Atkinson.

T.W Atkinson is mentioned in Edward Keith's book written in 1937 who was head gardener at Wallington Hall between 1882 and 1933, as follows:

> *"I never underwent a pulling by the Master (Isaac), but I did by his understudy, now defunct, and succeeded by his son, Mr Atkinson. We were pulling out the laurel stumps on the portico walk previous to planting the specimen conifers which still stand there. In falling back over I had slipped the main thigh muscle or tendon. For some fortnight I suffered untold agonies as I went about my work, the doctor whom I had consulted, saying it was muscular rheumatism and that I was to keep going about. As the pain got worse I slipped down to Morpeth (to see Mr Atkinson) unbeknown to the Mirlaw House expert (this is a property a few miles south of Wallington Hall where I guess his doctor lived) and two days later I was all right. After that I had little pity for the dislocated rabbits and howling dogs which had taught*

> *Milburn more than a Harley Street specialist ever knew. If ever a man deserved a tablet placed on the Town Hall of Morpeth to his memory it was Isaac Milburn. But there ! His studies begun and ended in the village school. How could he possibly know anything about the human frame? Impossible, absurd, a charlatan."*

It would appear that both of Atkinson's sons followed in the footsteps of their father as bonesetters. Charles Atkinson Bonesetter was advertising his services as an "Expert in Massage Work and Manipulative Surgery" from his home in Heaton Park Road, Heaton, Newcastle - daily 10 to 1 and 5 to 7 except Mondays. He also held weekly consultations at "The Grapes" Hotel, South Shields, "Ye Old 100" Hotel North Shields, "The Old White Swan", Cloth Market, Newcastle and "The Globe Inn" Clayton Street, Newcastle.

His other son Edward was also placing adverts as a bonesetter consulting at the following places:

Every Monday from 2 till 5 pm at T.Quinns, Railway Hotel, Blyth.

Every Wednesday & Saturday from 11 till 2, at Jos Clarks's, Black Bull Hotel, Bridge Street, Morpeth. (side entrance)

Every Pay Friday from 2 to 5, at Anderson's Café, 98, Station Road, Ashington (opposite Harmonic Hall)

Interestingly, one of Isaac's oldest living descendant's, Madge Galloway, nee Milburn, three times great granddaughter is 90 years old at the time I'm writing (April 2021) and now lives near Lincoln. Madge can recall travelling some distance from the Wooler area to Heaton, an area to the east of Newcastle city centre, after injuring herself as a young child by falling off a haystack in the 1930s and receiving treatment from Atkinson junior with the father T.W Atkinson present.

And so the bone-setting occupation continued in the 1930s much as it had done a hundred years earlier by receiving patients at the bonesetters residence and regular weekly surgeries in pubs.

Milburn's Oil

It was known that Isaac studied the herbs and plants in the countryside and made them up into oils and ointments which were widely used. A lady from Dunstan that Mary Kipling met during her researches had in her possession one of his prescription books which would be really interesting to read but I have been unable to track down. It included proverbs, the price of wheat over a number of years, and medical prescriptions for man and beast.

On Friday 17th March 1939 an advert appears in the Morpeth Herald which reads as follows

Milburns Oil

Prepared from the original recipe of the late Isaac Milburn Bonesetter and used as a massage oil for stiff joints, sprains, and muscle troubles

In bottles 1/3 and 1/6 by post 1/6 and 2/11

A.G.Marshall MPS

Pharmacist

43 & 45 Bridge St, Morpeth

Phone 227

MPS stands for Member of the Pharmaceutical Society and pricing is pre UK decimal; 1/3 is one shilling and three pennies. There were twelve pennies in a shilling and a shilling in 2020 is the same as 5 new pence in UK currency.

Isaac Milburn Statue

Sometime between 1888 and 1898 a statue figure of Isaac in a sitting position was exhibited in the window of George Rutherford and Sons, Drapers, Morpeth. It was then moved to a place in the garden of Mr Rutherford's residence in Dacre Street where it was still standing in 1928 "surrounded and surmounted by lichen and ivy a reminder of the ravages of time" according to a newspaper article of the time. In 1968 the Morpeth County Librarian, George Laughton, had assembled a small display of pictures and written material in the branch entrance about Isaac. My Milburn grandparents from Tweedmouth were approached with a view to loaning the original testimonial oil painting for the library display but declined as they feared it may be damaged or lost !!

Mr Laughton was keen to trace the whereabouts of the statue carved in stone by the firm of Henry Dobson and Sons of West Thirston near Felton. The missing sculpture has never been found and I wonder if it is still out there or has it been destroyed. Another question that comes to mind is why would a draper have this on display in his window and then move it into his garden? My first thoughts were was he a relative or possibly a patient? Maybe Isaac was considered a famous customer and this was the draper's way of showing respect to him after his death. It would certainly be an expensive exercise to commission a carved stone statue although Mr Rutherford was obviously a man of means with a thriving business allowing him to live in a substantial property called "Ash Trees" in Dacre Street. According to the 1891 census he was living there with his wife, ten children, one grandchild and two servants. The property still stands today and uses the same house name.

One of Isaac's relatives presented an oil painting of him to the Morpeth Library reference room in the late 1960s where it hung for a number of years. It was a copy of Isaac's testimonial painting by an unknown artist. Ironically I believe this ended up for sale not far from the Nags Head pub, in an antiques shop, a few years ago in Alnwick. A distant relative informed my uncle about the painting and by the time I found out and made enquiries the painting had been sold. Fortunately, the antiques dealer still had the contact details of the new owner and I was able to make an arrangement to purchase the painting.

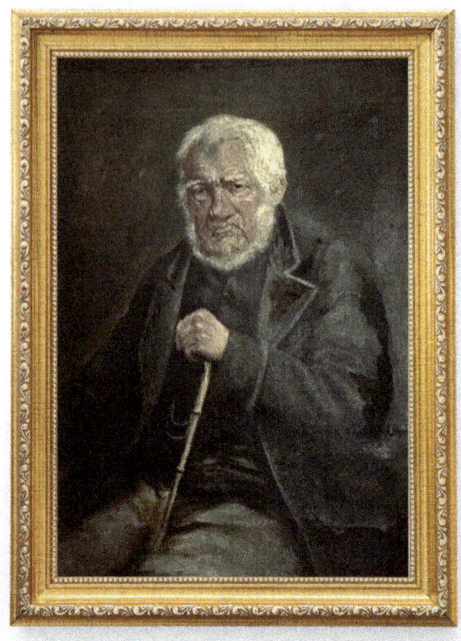

31. Oil painting

At the time when the painting was hanging in the Morpeth library, there were two framed texts, one a brief description of Isaac and his work, the other a poem about the old man by an anonymous author. Isaac treated many people of wealth, but his main concern was for the poor. As the poem recalls:

> "Tho' rough in speech in manner rude,
> With no deceit or shameful mood.
> His honest heart was true and good
> And to the end,
> With purse in hand, he always stood
> The poor man's friend."

We also know Isaac had an ear for music and made Northumbrian pipes. His handcrafting skills also extended to a walking stick carved from a holly branch with the handle in the shape of a human foot. He also made a carved needlework box for one of his relatives.

Mary Kipling also notes that although Isaac did not attend any particular church, he was a deeply religious man, reading his Bible, writing his own comments on the well-thumbed margins of each page. When he was ready to begin his day's work, he would go outside and, doffing his cap, would look heavenward, and ask for God's help and guidance to see him through the day.

His life was a most remarkable one, especially when one recalls his humble beginning and what he achieved by sheer determination and hard work, which included teaching himself to read and write.

The only physical reminders of Isaac's life that I know exist are the oil painting and his headstone. Hence this booklet of his life which will serve to preserve his life's work in print.

It would be wonderful if more family connections, a missing artifact or more tales turn up as a result of this publication.

"He possessed a genuine sympathy for his fellow men and many people in days gone past, have had reason to be grateful to that grand old man, Isaac Milburn.

May his memory live on." Mary Kipling

CHAPTER 10
MILBURN FAMILY TREE

32.

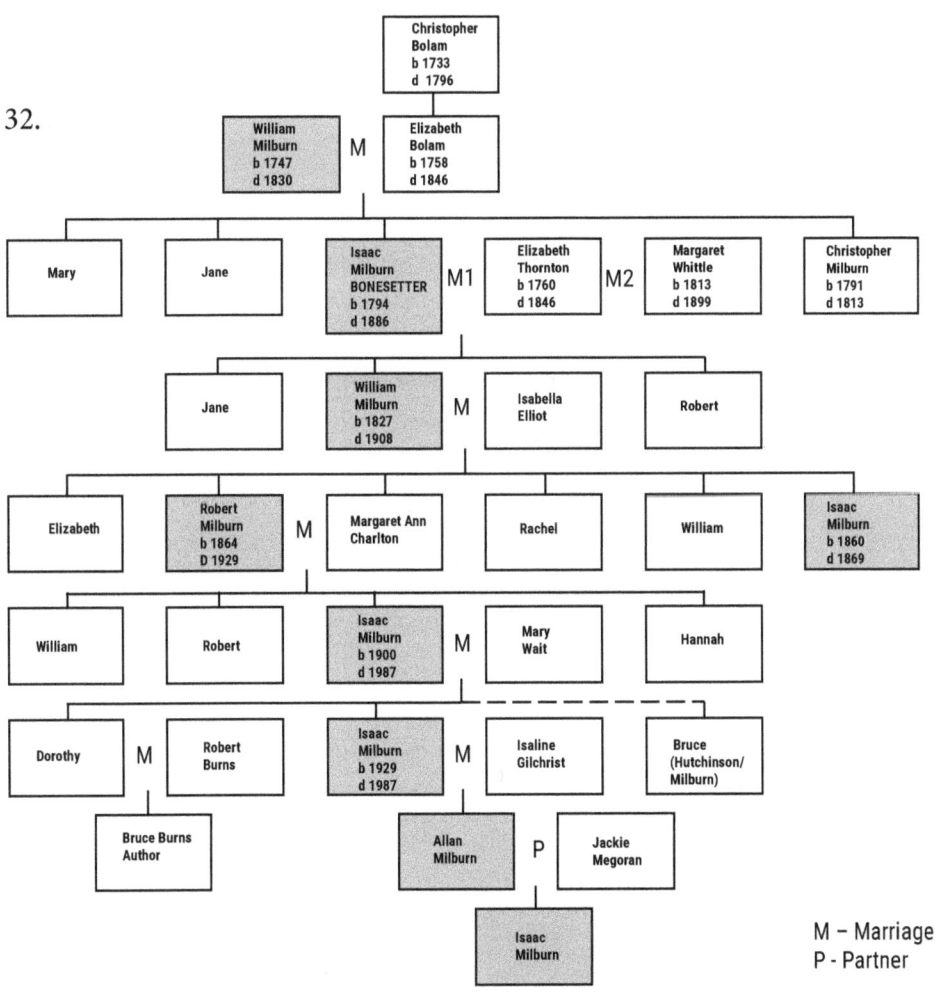

The earliest member I can find on Isaac's tree is his grandfather a Christopher Bolam born in 1733.

I have narrowed the tree down to show my closest lineage and how the name of Isaac has remained in this section of the Milburn family. There will undoubtedly be other Isaacs that have carried on in other lines but that would be a mammoth job to work out on another occasion. Isaac's name was first passed onto his grandson who was born in 1860 but sadly died in 1869.

The earliest Milburn photograph I have after Isaac the bonesetter is another grandson Robert Milburn born 1864.

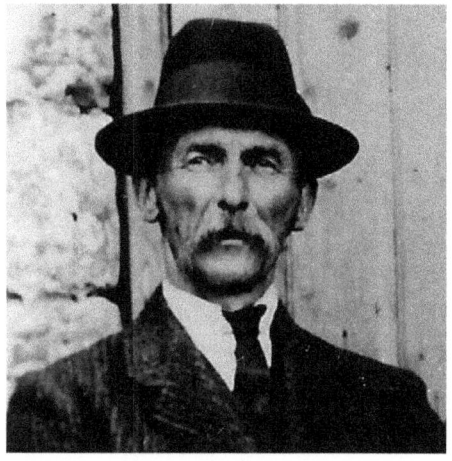

33. Robert Milburn.

Robert Milburn was working as a rabbit catcher at Newham, Northumberland in 1901.

Eventually he moved with his family to Sunnyside House Tweedmouth and it's said that he looked after and cut the nearby bowling club green in Spittal with a scythe - an agricultural implement with a long curved blade.

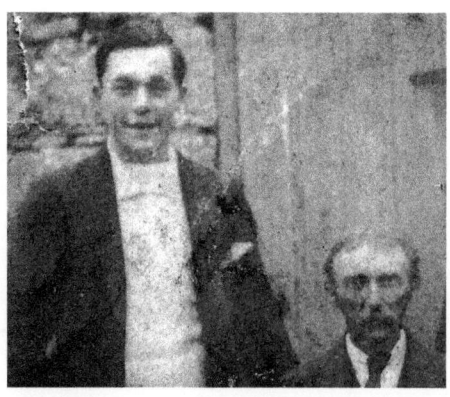

34. An early photo of great grandson Isaac Milburn born 1900 and his father Robert.

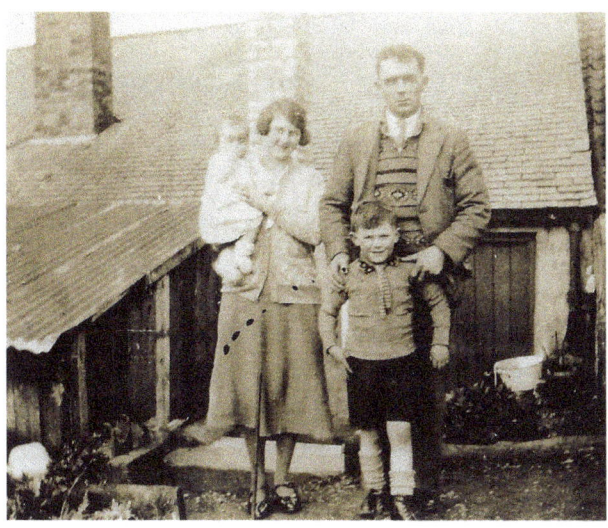

35. Great great grandson Isaac Milburn born 1929 is the young lad in front of his father his mother Mary and sister Dorothy – photo taken about 1935.

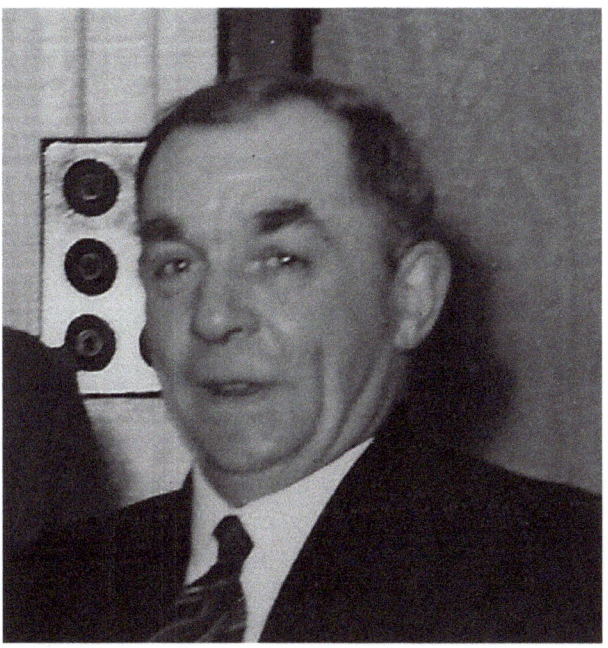

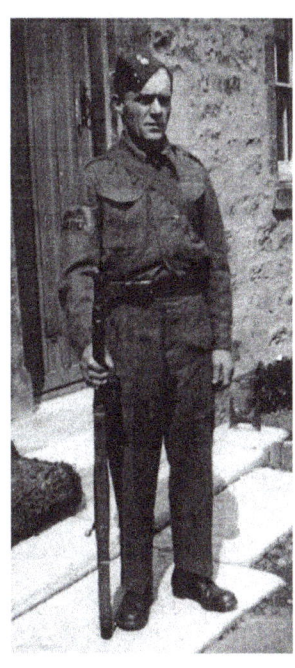

Isaac Milburn (photo 36), born 1900 photograph taken about 1960 worked for the COOP (the Cooperative Society) as a driver most of his working life and lived at Milburn House Tweedmouth. He volunteered as a fire warden during World War 2 at Tweedmouth East primary school on Mount Road. His twin brother Robert worked as a gamekeeper and lived at Ink Bottle Lodge near Greenlaw. He is pictured in his Alnwick home guard uniform during World War 2 (photo 37).

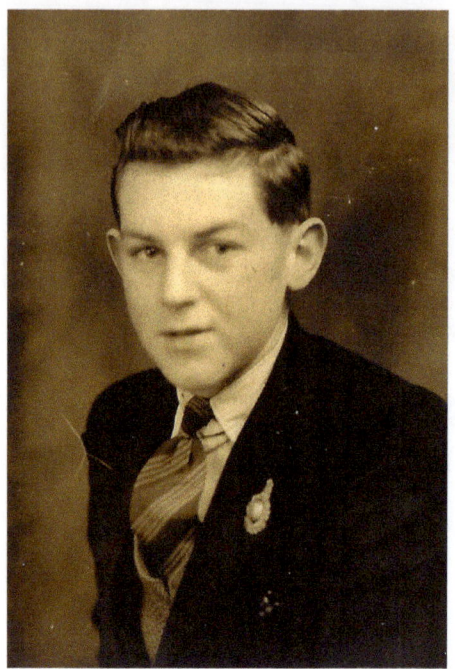
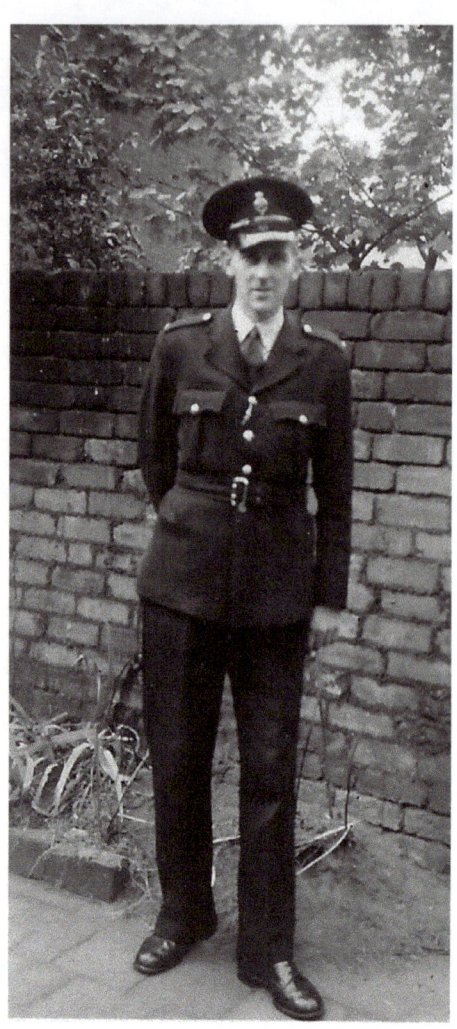

38 / 39. Isaac Milburn born 1929. Served his time as joiner at Allan Brothers Woodyard Tweedmouth then became a prison officer at both Liverpool and Durham jails.

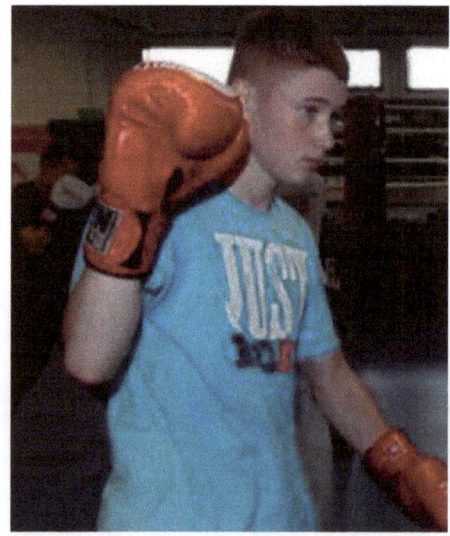

40. The name of Isaac continues to this day with Isaac Milburn born 1997 who was a top award-winning junior and senior boxer at Birtley Boxing Club where he fought at light welter weight for the Great Britain boxing team.

CHAPTER 11
KEY DATES

THOPHILL - WALLINGTON - 52 years		
Age	Year	Event
	1794	Born 6th April at Throphill near Mitford Northumberland.
29	1823	Married Elizabeth Thornton on the 12th April.
30	1824	Daughter Jane born. Baptised 5th March. Living at Bolt Cottage, Dovecot, Wallington Hall.
33	1827	Son William born.
35	1829	Swan tale.
36	1830	Smuggler's incident.
36	1830	13th October death of his father William age 83.
39	1833	Poaching tales.
42	1836	Son Robert born.
47	1841	Census living at Dovecot with wife Elizabeth, three children and working at Wallington Hall as a gamekeeper.
ELSDON - LONGFRAMLINGTON - 12 years		
Age	Year	Event
52	1846	Moved from Wallington Hall to Elsdon to work as a publican.
52	1846	23rd March - dinner with William Brewis at Thornton farm.
52	1846	Worked at Brinkburn as a Gamekeeper.

Age	Year	Event
52	1846	Moved to Longframlington and working as a publican at the Rimside Moor House Inn.
52	1846	15th May - first adverts offering bonesetting consultancy at the Bluebell Inn Alnwick and Goat Inn Cloth Market Newcastle.
52	1846	Elizabeth his mother died at Throphill age 88.
53	1847	Presented with a silver tea service.
57	1851	Census living with wife Elizabeth, three children in Longframlinton and working as a bonesetter.
60	1854	Marriage of daughter Jane at Framlington to William Leighton.

LONGHOUGHTON - 28 years

Age	Year	Event
63	1857	Death of wife Elizabeth Dec 1st.
64	1858	Jan 1st moved to Dusheugh near Alnwick. First grandchild born Elizabeth at Embleton.
67	1861	Census living alone at Dunsheugh, near Longhoughton - occupation bonesetter.
70	1864	Married second wife Margaret Whittle age 57 at Rennington church on the 24th Feb. Living at Drive Cottage, Longbank, Longhoughton.
70	1864	Exact date unknown – visited Buckingham Palace.
71	1865	Renting a garden beside Drive Cottage at the old Tile Works Longhoughton.
77	1871	Census living in Longhoughton with wife Margaret.
79	1873	Sanitary survey – invalided at the time.
86	1879	Testimonial and public dinner at the Nags Head Alnwick.
88	1881	Census living at Drive Cottage, Tile Sheds Longbank, Longhoughton with wife Margaret.
91	1885	Last bone setting advert 4th April working from home at Longbank age 91.
92	1886	Died 30th January age 92. His second wife Margaret died 13 years later age 86.

CHAPTER 12
SURNAME CAST LIST

Name	Occupation	Location
A		
Allan Ed		Alnwick
Anderson Thomas	Bonesetter	Winlanton
Archbald Joseph		
Atkinson Charles	Bonesetter	Heaton
Atkinson Edward B	Bonesetter	Morpeth
Atkinson Mr T.W	Bonesetter	Morpeth
B		
Bayley J Mr	Justice of the Peace	
Bell John		Alnwick
Bell Mat	Shooter	
Bell W		Alnwick
Black John	Farmer	Wooler
Blackett Kit Mr		
Bosanquet Miss	Ship passenger	
Brandling Charles	Magistrate	
Brewis William	Farmer/High Constable	Throphill

Name	Occupation	Location
Brown John		
Brown Miss	Publican	Newcastle
C		
Cadogan Hodgson	Estate Owner	Brinkburn
Chambers William	Doctor	Edinburgh
Charles	Servant	Wallington Hall
Charlton Mr		Wallington Hall
Clark Fergus	Publican	Alnwick
Cockburn Mr A.S		
Cockburn Mr Jos J		Alnwick
Codling Mr		Wallington Hall
Cookson	Estate owner	
Cooley Reverend W.L.J	Minister	
Cooper Mr	Exciseman	Wallington Hall
Crowther John	Bonesetter	Yorkshire
D		
Davidson A		Golden Moor farm Alnwick
Decies Lord	Ship passenger	
Dickson Mr	Steward	Mantle Hill
Dobson Henry	Sculptor	Thirston
Dodds Mr		Longhoughton
Donkin Robert		Rothbury
Dunn Miss	Publican	Alnwick
E		
Embleton Thomas	Auctioneer	Berwick
Evans Mr	Exciseman	

Name	Occupation	Location
G		
Galloway Madge	3 x great granddaughter	Lincoln
Gow Mr	Estate Manager	Wallington Hall
Gray Thos		Harlow Hill
Grey James		Low Stead Lesbury
Grey Mr R.T	Lambtons Bank employee	Alnwick
Griffiths Mr	Exciseman	Alnwick
H		
Hall William	Publican/brewer	Newcastle
Hawdon Mr	Surgeon	
Heddon John	Publican	Morpeth
Hickley John	Photographer	Alnwick
Horsley Jas		Alnwick
J		
Jeaffreson Christopher S	Surgeon	Newcastle
K		
Keith Edward	Head Gardener Writer	Wallington Hall
Kennedy William	Whisky Smuggler	
Kipling Mary	Artist / Writer	Consett
L		
Laughton George	Librarian	Morpeth
Lawes John	Servant	Wallington Hall
Leighton Mr W		Thirsleyhaugh
Liddle Edward		Gateshead

Name	Occupation	Location
Luke A Mrs	Isaac's great granddaughter	Hedley on the Hill
Lynn Mr	Patient	Shaftoe
M		
Main Alex Jas	Doctor	
Marshall Mr A.G	Pharmacist	Morpeth
Marshall John	Photographer / Artist	Alnwick
Mayor of Morpeth The		
McMillan Daniel	Sculptor	Alnwick
Milburn Elizabeth nee Thornton	Wallington Hall	
Milburn Jane		Wallington Hall
Milburn Margaret nee Whittle	Longhoughton	
Milburn Robert		Wallington Hall
Milburn William jnr		Wallington Hall
Milburn William snr	Cartwright	Throphill
Moore George	Draper	
N		
Newstead Jno	Court administrator	
O		
O'Hara Peter	Whisky Smuggler	
Orr Mr	Servant	Wallington Hall
P		
Percy Algernon George	6th Duke of Northumberland	Alnwick
Percy George	5th Duke of Northumberland	Alnwick

Name	Occupation	Location
Pott Mr	Servant	Wallington Hall
Princess Alexandra of Denmark	Princess of Wales	
Princess Beatrice		
Q		
Queen Victoria		
R		
Redman Mr		
Richardson Mr		Wallington Hall
Richardson Moses Aaron	Writer	
Riddell Mr Jas		Alnwick
Robertson Adam		Alnwick
Robinson George	Blacksmith	Longhoughton
Robinson William	Blacksmith	Longhoughton
Routledge Mr J	Publican	Consett
Rowantree John	Journalist	
Rutherford George	Draper	Morpeth
S		
Smailes Mr	Doctor	
Storey Mr	Bonesetter	Deckham
Stott Joe	Game Watcher	Harwood
Swinburne John Sir	Magistrate	Capheaton Hall
T		
Thomson Mr P		Alnwick
Thornton Jane	Isaacs mother-in-law	Wallington Hall
Trevelyan Catherine Anne Nee Forster	Wallington Hall	

Name	Occupation	Location
Trevelyan Edward Spencer		Wallington Hall
Trevelyan Maria Jane		
Trevelyan Sir George Otto	2nd Baronet	Wallington Hall
Trevelyan Sir John	4th Baronet	Wallington Hall
Trevelyan Sir John	5th Baronet	Wallington Hall
W		
Walsh Mrs	Cook	Wallington Hall
Wardle Elizabeth	Publican	Longframlington
Wardle John	Publican	Longframlington
Waterton Charles	Traveller and Naturalist	Wakefield
Weight Mrs	Bonesetter	Newcastle
Wilkinson Mr	Servant	Wallington Hall
Wilkinson Mr R	Woods & Co - Shop owner	Morpeth
Winship Mr	Servant	Wallington Hall

CHAPTER 13
PRINT REFERENCES

1. The Legend of Isaac Milburn/Legends of the North – Mary Kipling. Publisher John Shotton. Whiton Printers Wembley.
2. The Local Historians Table book of Remarkable Occurrences Vol 4 by Moses Aaron Richardson
3. Memories of Wallington Hall – Edward Keith 1937. Printed in GB by Purnell & Sons Ltd. (T.U) Paulton (Somerset) and London ASIN B0008C7404.
4. Isaac Milburn Bonesetter – Newcastle Courant Biography reprint from 28th March1879. Spottiswood and Co Printers London.
5. Frank Graham – Smugglers, Poachers and Bonesetters at Wallington Hall. ISBN 0859831264
6. Rosemary Muge (2018) Poverty, protest and sport: poaching in the East Midlands c.1820-1900. PhD thesis, University of Nottingham. http://eprints.nottingham.ac.uk/49161/1/Merged%20Whole%20Thesis%20Passed.pdf
7. The Diaries of William Brewis of Mitford 1833-1850 ISBN978-0-9538443-8-2. Published by Wagtail Press Hexham.
8. Brewers and Bottlers of Newcastle upon Tyne from 1850 to the present day. Brian Bennison, 1995,
9. The Diary of John Black 1863. Ford Westfield Farm. Ford. Northumberland. Unpublished.
10. Northumberland Gazette John Rowantree 1967
11. Queen Alexandra (London: Constable) ISBN 0-09-456560-0 Georgina Battiscombe 1968
12. The Shields Daily News 28th May 1887

Every effort has been made to trace copyright holders and to obtain their permission for the use of copyright material. The author apologizes for any errors or omissions in the above list and following image acknowledgements. He would be grateful if notified of any corrections that could be incorporated in future reprints or editions of this book.

CHAPTER 14
IMAGE ACKNOWLEDGEMENTS

Inside front cover	Map of Northumberland. Judith Yarrow.
1	Workshop. Courtesy of Northumberland Gazette, Nov 1967 / Bruce Burns
2	Restored property in 2021. Bruce Burns.
3	Wallington Hall. Bruce Burns.
4a / 4b	Bolt Cottage. Bruce Burns.
5	Edward Spencer Trevelyan. images@nationaltrust.org.uk under license.
6	Smugglers Map. Judith Yarrow.
7	Shaftoe Crags. Bruce Burns.
8	Frank Graham letter. Smugglers, Poachers and Bonesetters at Wallington Hall. ISBN 0859831264.
9	Notice. Courtesy of Newcastle Courant, 19th May 1854.
10a / 10b	Nags Head, Alnwick. Northumberland Archives NRO 9703/01.
11a / 11b	The Black Bull, Morpeth. Unknown / Bruce Burns.
12	Drive Cottage Map. Courtesy of Ordnance Survey.
13	Drive Cottage. Madge Galloway.

14	Drive Cottage. Courtesy of Northumberland Gazette Nov 1967.
15	Morpeth market. Late 1800s. Unknown.
16	Windy Gyle. Courtesy of Shepherds Walks.
17	Wooler and Windy Gyle distances map to Alnwick. Judith Yarrow.
18	Royal Command. Madge Galloway.
19	Queen Victoria Princess Beatrice. Royal Collection Trust / © Her Majesty Queen Elizabeth II 2020. RCIN 2900649.
20	Princess Alexandra 1863. Royal Collection Trust / © Her Majesty Queen Elizabeth II 2020.
21	Princess Alexandra + Queen Victoria. Royal Collection Trust / © Her Majesty Queen Elizabeth II 2020.
22	Longhoughton map. Courtesy of Ordnance Survey.
23	Drive Cottage map. Courtesy of Ordnance Survey.
24	Isaac Oil Portrait - also on front cover. John Marshall - Alnwick.
25	St Peter and St Paul Church map. Judith Yarrow.
26	Headstone. Bruce Burns.
27	St Peter and St Paul Church south/east view. Bruce Burns.
28	Painting. Mary Kipling.
29	Mary Kipling painting outside. Unknown
30	1881 Census record. imagelicensing@nationalarchives.gov.uk under license.
31	Oil painting. Unknown artist.
32	Family tree. Bruce Burns.
33 - 39	Family album photos.
40	Isaac Milburn boxing. NCJ Media Ltd.
41	The Author. Bruce Burns

IMAGE ACKNOWLEDGEMENTS

Inside back cover, 42	Royal Border Bridge between Tweedmouth and Berwick. Tommy McLeod Photography. t.mcleod@hotmail.com 07708 841145.
Inside back cover, 43	Alnwick Castle. Tommy McLeod Photography.
Inside back cover, 44	Shaftoe Crags. Bruce Burns.
Inside back cover, 45	Nature. Rachel Burns.
Inside back cover, 46	Cheviots. Jim Gibson Photography & Video Production. www.jimgibsonphotography.co.uk.
Inside back cover, 47a / 47b	Wallington Hall - entrance/coach house/stables. Bruce Burns.
Inside back cover, 48	Inside back cover. Morpeth clock tower. Bruce Burns.
Back cover	Painting by Mary Kipling.

CHAPTER 15
GLOSSARY

Aesculapius	a hero and god of medicine in ancient Greek religion and mythology
apocryphal	a story or statement of doubtful authenticity, although widely circulated as being true
attainted	to condemn by a sentence
aye	yes
bairn	child
baronet	a title that can be inherited but is not included in the order of nobility.
canna	cannot
canny	nice
cartwright	a maker of cartwheels
chaise	sometimes pronounced chay or shay, is a light two- or four-wheeled traveling or pleasure carriage for one or two people with a folding hood
de mortuus nil nisi bonum	of the dead, [say] nothing but good
diachylum	a type of adhesive plaster, formerly made of various plant juices, but later containing lead oxide and glycerine

drovers	men that walked sheep and cattle to market over long distances
duds	working clothes.
dye ye	do you
dyeun	done
fomented	bathed
frae	from
gan	go
Gaol	jail
gig	a two wheeled sprung single horse carriage
git	get
hirpled	walked about with a limp
humbler	possibly meaning degrading oneself by lying
hyem	home
jist	just
ken	knowledge
leader	medical term
luggish	whimp
noo	now
ocular	perceived
panegyric	a published text in praise of someone
mutch	a linen cap worn by older women
plaister	plaster powder and bandages
quack	one who falsely claims knowledge or skill of medicine
respited	reprieved
salts and senna	medicine made from minerals and herbs
secundum artem	a medical term meaning to use skill and judgement
shewn	shown

suppurating	producing a pus or festering
thee	you
tho	though
twitted	teased in jest
wa'alk	walk
watchers	lookouts for poachers
wi ya	with you
wise	way or manner
withal	in addition
wrought on	to persevere and continue to try and achieve an outcome
ye	you

ISAAC MILBURN: THE NORTHUMBRIAN BONESETTER 1794 - 1886

THE AUTHOR

Bruce was born in Berwick-Upon-Tweed where his father Robbie was a printer with the Berwick Advertiser and his mother trained as a weaver at Lords Mount Mill Berwick.

He was educated at Berwick Grammar School and then went on to graduate in Business Studies at the University of Bradford and represented the rowing team.

Bruce has never lost links with his hometown and his native Northumberland. He spent most of his school summer holidays working with his uncle and friends at the salmon fishing on the River Tweed, then a thriving industry. He supports Berwick Rangers, Newcastle United and the Scotland rugby team and is a regular spectator at Murrayfield.

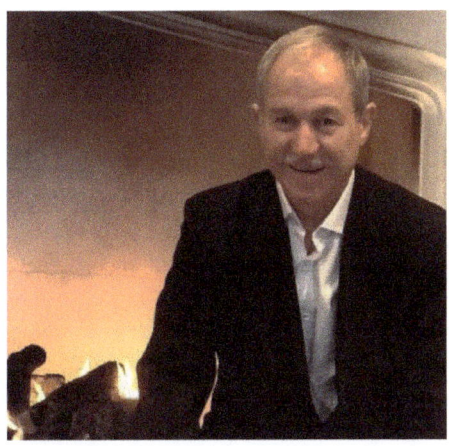

41. Bruce Burns.

He is keen on researching his family history and this book is an example of many hours of detailed work.

Bruce, who is also a thriving beekeeper, lives just outside Perth and travels up and down Scotland in the higher education audio visual business as a successful account manager.

www.ingramcontent.com/pod-product-compliance
Lightning Source LLC
Chambersburg PA
CBHW060924170426
43192CB00021B/2859